The Ethics of Coercion in
Mass Casualty Medicine

The Ethics of Coercion in Mass Casualty Medicine

GRIFFIN TROTTER, M.D., PH.D.
Associate Professor
Center for Health Care Ethics
Saint Louis University
Saint Louis, Missouri

The Johns Hopkins University Press
Baltimore

© 2007 The Johns Hopkins University Press
All rights reserved. Published 2007
Printed in the United States of America on acid-free paper
2   4   6   8   9   7   5   3   1

The Johns Hopkins University Press
2715 North Charles Street
Baltimore, Maryland 21218-4363
www.press.jhu.edu

Library of Congress Cataloging-in-Publication Data

Trotter, Griffin, 1957–
The ethics of coercion in mass casualty medicine / Griffin Trotter.
p. ; cm.
Includes bibliographical references and index.
ISBN-13: 978-0-8018-8551-8 (hardcover : alk. paper)
ISBN-10: 0-8018-8551-5 (hardcover : alk. paper)
1. Emergency medical services—Moral and ethical aspects. 2. Mass
casualties—Moral and ethical aspects. 3. Disaster relief—Moral and
ethical aspects. I. Title.
[DNLM: 1. Coercion. 2. Public Health Practice—ethics. 3. Disasters.
4. Emergency Treatment—ethics. 5. Health Policy. 6. Patient Rights—
ethics. 7. Terrorism. WA 525 T858e 2007]
RA645.5.T76 2007
174'.936218—dc22   2006017420

A catalog record for this book is available from the British Library.

Contents

Preface

This book inquires about coercion in mass casualty medicine: What are its proposed uses? How are these justified? Which justifications are adequate? The term *coercion* here denotes the intentional use of a credible and severe threat of harm or force to control others. *Mass casualty medicine* denotes preparation for and provision of medical treatment or other health-preserving actions in mass casualty events or in situations in which large numbers of casualties will result unless there is quick and decisive intervention. Much of the preparation and implementation in mass casualty medicine (MCM), including proposed uses of coercion, occurs at the level of public policy and public health oversight. Hence, this book deals not only with clinical mass casualty medicine, in which medical services are rendered directly to victims, but also, and perhaps more importantly, with public policy and public health issues. Indeed, public deliberation about uses of coercion in MCM occurs predominantly at the policy-making level. When rescuers and clinicians encounter victims in the field, there is little time for individual deliberation—and the time for public deliberation typically has passed.

Mass casualty events occur when large numbers of serious casualties (i.e., seriously injured or ill individuals), usually ranging in the thousands, generate overwhelming demands on local health care systems. Coercion is used in MCM when it is crucial that the public, or one of its subgroups, comply with directives that they cannot be trusted to follow voluntarily. Possible examples are (1) forced isolation and quarantine of ill or exposed individuals, (2) conscription of health care workers for service in MCM, (3) physical detainment of individuals who need to be decontaminated after a chemical or radiological exposure, (4) forced medical treatment or examination, (5) legal sanctions against those who attempt to acquire or distribute restricted medical treatments (such as the smallpox immunization), and (6) legal sanctions against those who publicly reveal restricted scientific information (such as the formula for a lethal chemical warfare agent). Each of these instances of coercion, and several others, are treated in this book.

The most common precipitants of mass casualty events are disasters such as hurricanes, earthquakes, tornadoes, chemical spills, explosions, nuclear events, and epidemics (though not all such disasters cause mass casualties). Among the most feared of these disasters are human-made, intentional disasters perpetrated, for instance, by terrorists wielding weapons of mass destruction. In the aftermath of the September 11 attacks and the subsequent anthrax attack in the United States, public concern over these threats is high, and there are large-scale efforts to develop workable prevention and response strategies. Hence, much of the discussion in this book focuses on intentional attacks and the complex political, public health, and medical structures that are emerging as we struggle to address them. On the other hand, the preparation for and response to natural disasters has hardly been perfected. As this book neared completion, Hurricane Katrina struck the Gulf Coast region of the United States, killing hundreds and causing massive social and economic damages—much of which was preventable, given better disaster preparations. A year earlier, warning systems proved inadequate as a tsunami in Asia produced far more staggering devastation. Hoping to preclude further debacles, politicians and other policy makers currently are spending billions of dollars to address the threat of a global avian influenza epidemic.

In the effort to prepare for these natural disasters, many of the same coercive strategies and tactics discussed in the context of intentional disasters are now being proposed. Indeed, the increasingly familiar notion of "all-hazards" disaster preparation draws from the overlapping content in strategies designed for intentional disasters and those designed for natural disasters. We will find in the ensuing discussion that many intentional disasters bear more in common with analogous natural disasters than with other intentional disasters. In the end, factors such as the appearance of warning signs, the timing and duration of effects, lethality, transmissibility, and the threat to social structures are what matter most in gauging our preparation and response. The distinction between intentional disasters, accidents, and natural disasters is less important.

Because this book focuses on crucial factors that pertain in the response to both intentional disasters and natural disasters, it should be useful for inquirers into both phenomena. It will also be of interest to readers with a general interest in public health ethics and/or public policy ethics, because coercion and its political legitimization are central to any discussion of these topics.

The book is written in a relatively nontechnical style so that it will be accessible to scholars, students, and practitioners from a multiplicity of academic and practical disciplines that address various aspects of mass casualty medicine and public health ethics. Case narratives are frequently used. When it is necessary to use technical terms and concepts, I have tried to define or characterize them in a manner that will assist readers who lack relevant technical training.

On the other hand, since the book purports to contribute to scholarship on disaster medicine, clinical ethics, public health ethics, and political philosophy, intricate argumentation and engagement with the scholarly literature are needed. Some of the material that will be of interest primarily to scholars is relegated to the notes. But throughout the text I have made an effort to maintain a depth of reasoning that will satisfy scholarly readers, including those with advanced training in ethics, political philosophy, disaster sociology, public health, and disaster medicine.

One of my objectives in writing this book is to produce a text that can be used in public health ethics courses. In this regard, the second chapter, "Public Health and Its Ethical Basis," provides a basic context for public health ethics, and the third chapter, "Legitimacy," provides much-needed theoretical underpinnings—both of which are difficult to find in the current literature on public health ethics. The sections in the third chapter addressing deliberative democracy, rational consensus, and modus vivendi theory are especially relevant for advanced students and scholars in bioethics and philosophy, and I am hoping that it will address critical needs for such readers. More casual readers may want to skim over these sections.

Mass casualty medicine is public medicine, implemented under harsh conditions. Municipal, state, and national bodies formulate strategies, collect and organize resources, and train practitioners—all with an eye to quick, coordinated, and efficient intervention. Forms of coercion that are normally out of bounds may be justified in MCM just because it demands such a high level of efficiency and integration. Prolonged deliberation, elaborate attempts at persuasion, and the indulgence of individual idiosyncrasy become unworkable. Large-scale cooperation is demanded for many diverse and disparately inclined citizens and groups. And sometimes coercion is needed to guarantee it.

In tension with this demand for unified action is the value of individual and group self-determination. Under normal conditions, public morality in pluralistic democracies like the United States dictates that self-determination is the more fundamental concern. Citizens decide for themselves when they need medical attention. They move about freely. They choose where and when they want to work. And they trade their goods and services with little impediment. In the context of mass casualty medicine, however, these liberties are typically abridged. The equilibrium between state authority and private prerogative shifts in the direction of the state.

As I discuss in chapter 1, this equilibrium shift is manifested at the level of both public policy and operations. At the policy level, it manifests in proposals such as the recent Model State Emergency Health Powers Act that seek to enhance the legal authority of the state to appropriate property and intrude on personal liberties in the service of public ends. At the level of operations, it manifests in a Rescue Paradigm (RP) that focuses strongly on the reduction of death and disability within the population as a whole. Standard mortality and morbidity parameters, rather than individual preferences, are used to measure success. Though the standardization of objectives is evident to some degree in ordinary patient-centered clinical medicine (OCM), it is far more pronounced in mass casualty medicine.

At a deeper level, the equilibrium between state authority and private prerogative represents a negotiated balance between two sometimes-opposed public values: security and liberty. The shift in emphasis toward state authority occurs when security is drastically threatened. From the standpoint of ethics and public policy, the critical issue is how to strike a legitimate new balance. The value of individual liberty, after all, does not evaporate in a public emergency.

Prescribing the proper proportionality between security and liberty is difficult under the best of circumstances. These conflicting values are, as the saying goes, like apples and oranges. They are not easily compared and contrasted. To balance them effectively, one needs a well-developed capacity of practical judgment or prudence. But the virtue of prudence is itself rather slippery. It is a function of moral vision. Prudent Viking warriors, for instance, think and behave differently than do prudent Roman Catholic monks.

In the context of mass casualty medicine, social cohesion is paramount. But cohesion is threatened by the diversity of moral visions — a diversity involving incompatible and incommensurable beliefs that manifest across the entire spectrum of moral thinking. At one end of the spectrum are contrasting visions of the metaphysics of morals. Do our values come from God, from reason, or from the laws of nature? Concern for such metaphysical conundrums will be attenuated in this study, though indeed, beliefs about these matters can sometimes affect the way various people respond to mass casualty threats. At the other, more immediately practical end of the spectrum are visions of professional, civic, and domestic morality. As illustrated in chapter 1, the civic values that inform prudent policy makers are likely to differ in important ways from the professional values that inform prudent public health officials and clinicians. Finally, because policy directives are ineradicably vague and ambiguous, they must be interpreted by the officials and clinicians who eventually enact them. As interpretations unfold, the new equilibrium between security and liberty that policy makers thought they were establishing is apt to shift once again.

Insofar as it represents the provisional moral outlook of clinicians in the field, the aforementioned Rescue Paradigm might be regarded as the clinical terminus in this chain of shifting equilibriums. Hence, the Rescue Paradigm should not be viewed as a whole new ethics of medicine. It is, more or less, the old ethics of medicine adapted to a new context—mass casualty medicine—reflecting a provisional new balance between the values of security and liberty. In like manner, emergency powers legislation does not prescribe new political principles. It employs the old array of principles, adapted to a dramatic but temporary new context. One of the keys to understanding policy decisions and professional decisions in mass casualty medicine, then, is to explore the underlying moral visions of policy makers, professionals, and the citizens they seek to serve. Chapter 1 briefly examines medical ethics and contrasts its manifestations in ordinary clinical medicine with those in rescue medicine. It also begins to develop the context for coercive decisions in MCM and initiates an examination of policy makers' values by (1) examining some of the aforementioned pitfalls in translating public directives into clinical decisions, (2) explaining the concept of coercion, (3) discussing the Model State Emergency Health Powers Act (MSEHPA), and (4) showing how diverging appraisals of MSEHPA hinge on diverging accounts of the operation of trust in MCM. While advocates of extensive emergency coercive powers tend to perceive government agents as largely trustworthy, and citizens (including, on some accounts, clinicians) as largely untrustworthy (and untrusting), opponents of state coercion tend to believe just the opposite.

Chapter 2 investigates general approaches to justifying coercion in public health. It begins by looking at the task of public health, noting that it is variously described as (1) assuring the conditions for good health; or (2) assuring, insofar as this is possible, good health itself. The perplexities that arise from these diverging interpretations of the office of public health are complicated by the fact that "health" is itself an elusive, value-laden concept.

Next we look at the alleged tension between individual interests and the common good, which is frequently offered as the fundamental moral problem for public health ethics. This description is rejected because the concept of "common good," on most accounts, consists largely of an aggregation of individual interests and rights (such that the prior formulation unhelpfully denotes tension between the common good and itself). I argue for an alternative account: that the primary problem for public health ethics is gauging the proper balance between security (from illness and injury) and liberty.

Public health systems, we note, are subsystems of the larger polis, which for its part also pursues other ends besides good health and its conditions. One moral pitfall in public health practice is the tendency to neglect or repudiate the subordinate status of public health subsystems and enshrine the public's health as a fundamental and overriding political value. This tendency constitutes a deleterious threat to legitimate moral pluralism in that it begets attempts to fashion a uniform definition and standard of health and that it subordinates politically crucial liberty values. Of course, the threat looms larger when public health authorities are granted special coercive powers. Chapter 2 concludes with a look at pre-theoretical approaches to the ethics of coercion in public health.

Chapter 3 shifts to more general questions about public policy, public morality, and their interface with the moral visions of individual citizens. It seeks to articulate the ethical basis for political legitimacy in intrusive state actions, including the basis for legitimate state actions that involve coercion. Two forms of legitimacy are frequently invoked. Good reasons legitimacy (GRL) consists in the existence of cogent arguments (good reasons) to justify the state's intrusion. Public justification legitimacy (PJL) consists in the operation of procedures for obtaining public input about proposed interventions or for informing the public about their rationale that are sufficient to the demands of democracy. Though good reasons legitimacy is frequently portrayed as the primary basis for political legitimacy, what counts as a good reason or a good argument typically hinges on public values. Hence, I argue that PJL is a more fundamental source of political authority than GRL in democratic societies (especially morally pluralistic ones) and is the key to articulating an account of political legitimacy. This thesis has been championed recently by the proponents of deliberative democracy.

The bulk of chapter 3 investigates two competing theories of authority in deliberative democracy: *rational consensus theory*, which aims at establishing moral consensus through rational public deliberation; and *modus vivendi theory*, which aims at establishing a peaceful compromise that enjoys the consent of contending parties. I argue for the latter on the basis that (1) it is truer to the actual nature of public deliberation, which is not a wholly rational affair; (2) it avoids morally imperialistic attempts to delineate the domain of "rational" discourse; (3) it recognizes the deep and refractory nature of certain moral controversies; (4) it preserves a more generous space for moral pluralism and also for moral inquiry by enacting strong standards of permission and consent; and (5) its focus on peaceful mediation acts as a counterweight against the forceful imposition of prematurely declared consensus. The chapter concludes with illustrations of the modus vivendi approach and its operation in mass casualty medicine. Several obstacles are noted, including questions about participation in public deliberation—its loci, epistemic warrants, and contexts—and about how applications of the modus vivendi approach in MCM might adapt to contextual features and idiosyncrasies that characterize particular mass casualty events. These questions provide the subject matter for subsequent chapters.

Chapter 4 examines the role of experts such as ethicists, public health specialists, clinicians, and scientists in public deliberation and policy formulation for MCM. It also looks, more briefly, at the role of the news media. These sources (experts and the news media) often act synergistically in providing public deliberators with information they need to fruitfully examine particular policy options. Experts about factual issues are also frequently employed as expert deliberators and policy formulators. In regard to the latter, expertise in various factual realms is often conflated with expertise about values and norms. However, even experts in ethics are not experts in delineating authoritative values. To the contrary, they are experts in describing systems of values and in explaining how they hold together. If public justification determines what counts as a good argument or good reasons (as chapter 3 argues), then the general public—not its experts—is the authoritative source of political values. In formulating evidence-based guidelines for mass casualty medicine, I suggest the employment of an evidence classification scheme that sorts out fact and value claims in accordance with their doxastic security. Fact claims are doxastically secure when they are strongly based on good evidence. Value claims are doxastically secure when they are not immediately vulnerable to revision or dispute. The proper role of experts will vary depending on the respective doxastic security of fact and value claims.

Decisions about coercion in mass casualty medicine can be roughly classified into four categories: (1) policy decisions (as in approving legislation or regulations), (2) strategic leadership decisions (as in ordering general interventions such as quarantine), (3) tactical leadership decisions (as in instructing police to secure the boundaries of a hot zone), and (4) decisions about particular actions (as in deciding that a patient needs to be isolated). Chapter 5 begins an inquiry about involvement in deliberation, specifically addressing policy decisions and strategic leadership. It asks: Who should have a right to input? Where does the authority for final decisions lie? and What sorts of constraints should apply to this authority? The answers to these questions will vary, I argue, depending on the context and on the basic rationale for intervention. One rationale for coercion in MCM is the prevention of self-harm (manifested, for instance, in legal restrictions against obtaining or distributing smallpox vaccines). I argue that the primary deliberators about actions that threaten self-harm should ideally be the affected agents themselves (for instance, the patient who is contemplating smallpox immunization). Nevertheless, certain contingencies (decision-making capacity inadequate for the given task; inadequate time to impart or assimilate relevant information) may justify the usurpation of this individual pre-rogative. The other two rationales for coercion are preventing harm to others (as in quarantine) and securing personnel and resources that are needed to help others (as in taking property). In each of these cases, there ought to be input from the affected public.

Because direct participation in deliberation is typically limited when large numbers are involved, it is necessary to use community leaders who can represent the interests of their constituency. Ideally, leaders from each affected moral community would be included. But the boundaries between various moral communities and their memberships are hard to delineate. As an approximation, geographic boundaries (neighborhoods, cities, states) are typically used to allot the sources of deliberative input. Though this surrogate is fraught with moral hazard, it tends to work fairly well in disaster planning, since disasters tend to be geographically well-focused and to evoke a partial coalescence of individual values. Techniques such as deliberative polling potentially help to ensure that there is broad representation from each particular moral enclave within a geographical unit such as a neighborhood or borough. At the level of national deliberation, state representation prevails (where representatives ideally introduce values established through broad deliberation within their jurisdictions). Much of chapter 5 investigates the distribution of authority between federal, state, and local officials. To a large degree, I argue, proper jurisdiction will depend on the characteristics of particular threats. As an aid in sorting out salient characteristics, a threat classification scheme is developed, and its implications for the distribution of authority are examined.

Chapter 6 investigates tactical leadership decisions to enact coercion in mass casualty medicine. Tactical decisions typically differ from policy decisions and strategic leadership decisions in that they allow little opportunity for group deliberation. Several barriers to good tactical decision making are elicited through an analysis of the events of 9/11. These include: (1) the operation of false dogmas and assumptions (particularly with regard to the occurrence and nature of emergent social action); (2) the operation of maladaptive protocols that centralize authority; and (3) inefficient information exchange. Much of the subsequent discussion focuses on how these barriers operate when coercion is employed or considered in various mass casualty situations. The Incident Command System (ICS) is examined and the "command-and-control" philosophy exhibited by many of its proponents is criticized (primarily for its failure to recognize and exploit emergent social action).

Tactical decisions are justified when they employ and integrate good reasons (reasons that ideally have a basis in prior public deliberation). With this feature in mind, chapter 6 concludes by enumerating several characteristics of good tactical leadership. These include (1) an ability to understand and interpret publicly issued guidelines in a manner that reflects the original intentions of those who framed them; (2) an understanding of relevant facts; (3) technical competence, ideally acquired through effective rehearsal and training; (4) adaptability (especially in considering alternatives to coercion, facilitating cooperation, and directing resources to areas of critical need); and (5) public responsiveness (to contributions from citizens, news media, and colleagues).

The final chapter examines the enactment of coercive decisions at the level of individual action. Police actions and the coercive actions of individual citizens are examined, followed by a more detailed analysis of the operation of coercion in clinical mass casualty medicine. Fundamental difficulties arise in balancing the clinician's usual focus on service to individual patients against an augmented responsibility to protect the public, and in dealing with the "Rescuer's Paradox"—that, on one hand, psychological detachment is necessary for efficiency and effectiveness under the harsh conditions that typify clinical MCM and, on the other hand, deep engagement with public motives and ends is necessary to sustain and direct the clinician's efforts. Ultimately, there is no alternative for the virtuous clinician but willingness to share partially in the suffering of the afflicted. Otherwise, the disaster victim becomes a disconnected "other"—and coercion is an exceedingly comfortable alternative in the management of "others."

Acknowledgments

Much of the groundwork for this book was laid during visits to specialized libraries and academic centers in the northeastern United States. Many of these visits occurred in the fall of 2004. I am grateful to Saint Louis University for a faculty research leave award that provided time and money for these travels and to Gerard Magill for facilitating the process. I also deeply appreciate the hospitality and expert advice from staff and faculty members at the Disaster Research Center at the University of Delaware during my 2004 visit. Russell Dynes, Havidán Rodríquez, Tricia Wachtendorf, and Benigno Aguirre all helped, though they should not be held accountable in any way for errors or other shortcomings in my text. At the University of Virginia, Jonathan Moreno was both a fabulous host and a crucially important dialogue partner in the brainstorming stage of this project.

H. Tristram Engelhardt Jr. read a draft of the third chapter and offered many helpful comments. He is an energetic, loyal mentor who is always available whenever I need help—even when the task involves criticizing his own work. The Johns Hopkins University Press provided an excellent anonymous reviewer, who contributed significantly to the quality of the book. The copyeditor, Elizabeth Yoder was, without question, the best I have worked with.

This book would never have been written if not for the foresight, patience, and expertise of Wendy Harris, acquisitions editor for the Johns Hopkins University Press. She is the consummate professional.

Many colleagues deserve recognition for their scholarly contributions and willingness to serve as dialogue partners, critics, and motivators. In addition to those noted above, the short list includes Thomasine Kushner, John Lachs, James DuBois, Mark Cherry, Ana Iltis, Sandy Johnson, Jill Burkemper, Lisa Eckenwiler, Shug McBay, Mark Kuczewski, Micah Hester, Kelly Parker, George Khushf, Fabrice Jotterand, Lisa Rasmussen, Arthur Anderson, Alex London, Felicia Cohn, Lawrence Gostin, George Annas, Mark Hall, Kenneth Kipnis, and Tom Koch.

The Ethics of Coercion in
Mass Casualty Medicine

CHAPTER ONE

The Dynamics of Coercion in Mass Casualty Medicine

Imagine that terrorists spray a concentrated *Francisella tularensis* aerosol into a large government office building in Dover, Delaware.[1] At t_0 (the time at which the microorganisms are released), there is no awareness of the impending tragedy, and the daily shuffle goes undisturbed. Three days later, dozens of persons from the building present to Dover clinics and emergency departments with severe pneumonia. The rapid influx of patients is identified by public health authorities, and suspicions of terrorism are aroused. Fluorescent antibody testing of several patients for tularemia (which takes about 2–3 hours) is positive, but strict confirmation by culture will require at least three to five days, perhaps even weeks. Epidemiologists quickly identify the office building as a likely source. They advise Delaware's governor that thousands more may be exposed and that other loci could have been seeded with the bacterium. Also noted is the fact that tularemia — even the inhalational form now apparently being observed — is not generally spread from person to person. The governor, in accordance with provisions of the Delaware Emergency Health Powers Act (DEHPA) encoded in Title 20, Chapter 32 of the Delaware Code, declares a public health emergency.

DEHPA is not fictional. It was introduced as House Bill 377 on March 20, 2002, by Delaware State Representative Maier. The initial language and content (drafted by Matthew Denn, an attorney in the governor's office) mostly recapitulated another document — the Model State Emergency Health Powers Act (MSEHPA), drafted at the behest of the Centers for Disease Control (CDC) by legal and public health scholars from the Center for Law and the Public's Health at Georgetown and Johns Hopkins Universities.[2] In deliberation over the Delaware legislation, seven amendments were proposed, and five approved.[3] The amended bill passed and was signed on July 3, 2002. Included in the bill are provisions, similar to those in MSEHPA, for the institution of isolation and quarantine during a public health emergency (the latter defined in terms drawn from MSEHPA).[4] Delaware legislators also eventually rejected certain elements of MSEHPA. For example, provisions enhancing public health authority to appropriate hospitals and certain other property and to deny licensure to uncooperative physicians were scratched from the original bill.

Let us return to the hypothetical tularemia attack.

Though there is a live attenuated vaccine for tularemia, it is not widely available in the United States, and its effectiveness in post-exposure prophylaxis is unproven.[5] Hence, Delaware officials identify antibiotics as the treatment of choice. Ill individuals are admitted for parenteral (intravenous) antibiotics, and attempts are made to locate other individuals who are likely to have been exposed and start them on treatment with oral doxycycline or ciprofloxacin.

A physician, Marcia Welby, encounters a patient who visited the government building briefly during the period in which the attack is thought to have occurred. The young woman has abruptly developed a high fever, headache, sore throat, and cough. She is severely allergic to quinolone antibiotics such as ciprofloxacin and refuses treatment with doxycycline because she is nursing a feeble, premature infant whose liver problems might be exacerbated by receiving the antibiotic through breast milk.[6] The patient says she is willing to take her chances with the disease (which untreated has a mortality of about 30%) rather than risk treatment for an illness she knows is not likely to be passed to her child. Dr. Welby notifies the public safety authority and recommends that the patient be isolated in a hospital until she accepts treatment.

Dr. Welby's explicit reasoning is that the patient poses a transmission risk to her infant. Though person-to-person transmission of tularemia is not documented,[7] experience is limited, and Dr. Welby proposes that this case may be one in which it could occur with catastrophic results for the infant. Dr. Welby notes that the virulence and transmissibility of the organism afflicting her patient are undetermined. It could be a weaponized bacterium, causing an illness with different transmission characteristics than ordinary tularemia. Furthermore, she points out, it is still possible that the agent is something other than *Francisella tularensis*. Police arrive at the clinic, and the patient is forcibly hospitalized. She capitulates and begins a course of antibiotics. Later, Dr. Welby reflects on this case with satisfaction. Though the likelihood of mother-to-infant transmission was extremely low, Dr. Welby's decision was consonant with the law (its explicit basis being the intention to prevent the spread of "possibly contagious disease"), and it may well have saved her patient's life. Saving lives, Dr. Welby believes, is the fundamental consideration that should drive clinical decisions in mass casualty medicine (MCM).

In this case, Dr. Welby and the public safety authority make a decision about the use of coercion. Their decision, in distinction to the Delaware legislation authorizing it, is highly clinically specific. In fact, Dr. Welby's decision and the legislators' decision illustrate opposite sides of a spectrum of possible decisions about the use of coercion in MCM. At one end of the spectrum are public policy decisions (as in the legislation) and strategic decisions; at the other end are tactical decisions and decisions for particular coercive actions (as in the hospitalization of the patient with suspected tularemia). Strategic decisions are general in nature. They are meant to apply in a wide variety of specific circumstances and tend to be relatively removed in time and space from their various applications. Tactical decisions are context-bound and are enacted in response to particular problems. Typically the interval between decision and enactment is brief, and the decision maker is imbedded in circumstances that necessitate the tactical decision.

THE CONTEXT OF MASS CASUALTY MEDICINE

As this hypothetical case illustrates, strategic and tactical decisions do not merge seamlessly. Strategic initiatives such as the health powers laws must be interpreted by public health officials, law enforcement officers, and clinicians—and the interpretations will vary, depending on the frame of reference of the interpreter. Hence, when strategic initiatives such as emergency powers laws are formulated, it is difficult to predict how they will be enacted.

The primary tools of interpretation are information (or "facts") and values. Information about specific events (such as the outbreak of respiratory illness in our example) provides conditions for enacting strategies (such as DEHPA) in particular tactical contexts. In mass casualty response, information trickles in irregularly. Sometimes it will be distressingly sparse, and sometimes it will be largely inaccurate. At the operations level, clinicians and rescuers process available information in a manner that reflects their training. Facts are arranged in patterns that reflect core values such as the imperative to save lives or the obligation to respect persons' decisional autonomy.

Sometimes, as in our tularemia scenario, certain values will be at odds. What sort of guarantee do we have that operations personnel will balance conflicting values in the way that strategists intend? To answer, one must ascertain how agents will translate strategic guidelines—as, for example, in specifying the limit of improbability where a "possibly contagious disease" becomes, for practical purposes, a nontransmissible one. Is the same limit applied by both strategists and tacticians?

In the tularemia scenario, our answer to the latter question is likely negative. It seems improbable that legislators writing guidelines for involuntary detention of victims of bioterrorism and epidemics would regard an outbreak of an illness such as tularemia, which has never been known to be transmitted, as sufficient stimulus for forced isolation. Isolation and quarantine amount to virtual imprisonment of the innocent, and that is simply too great an infringement for publicly beholden representatives to countenance without a serious transmission threat. But Dr. Welby appealed to a different hierarchy of values. In her mind, the overwhelming consideration was saving lives. Legislative guidelines were viewed through the lens of this supreme value. Though the preservation of liberty is arguably government's primary ethical mandate,[8] Dr. Welby's personal values and professional training led her to focus on a different mandate. To understand this perspective and how it operates generally, it is useful to examine the ethical paradigm that animates clinicians and rescuers in mass casualty medicine.

THE RESCUE PARADIGM

A mass casualty event is an occurrence that produces large numbers of serious casualties (i.e., seriously injured or ill individuals), usually ranging in the thousands, such that the burden on health care systems in the locality of the occurrence becomes many times greater than usual. Mass casualty events should be differentiated from disasters. The former are marked by the large number of casualties and the resulting mismatch between medical needs and immediate medical capabilities. Health care professionals sometimes define disasters in such terms. For instance, the American College of Emergency Physicians defines a medical disaster as an occurrence in which "the destructive effects of natural or manmade forces overwhelm the ability of a given area or community to meet the demand for health care."[9] But seasoned disaster researchers tend to define disasters in terms of social disruptions. Thus, for instance, Fritz defines a *disaster* as "an event, concentrated in time and space, in which a society, or a relatively self-sufficient subdivision of society, undergoes severe danger and incurs such losses to its members and physical appurtenances that the social structure is disrupted and the fulfillment of all or some of the essential functions of the society is prevented."[10] Some of these researchers also employ another term, *catastrophe*, for extremely large-scale disasters. In a catastrophe, as opposed to an ordinary disaster, most or all of a community's structure is affected, such that displaced victims are unable to seek shelter with nearby relatives, and local officials are unable to undertake their usual duties (sometimes for prolonged periods).[11] Hurricane Katrina's impact in parts of Louisiana and Mississippi is an example of a catastrophe. Of course, many disasters and catastrophes are mass casualty events, and most mass casualty events are disasters.[12] Hence, in much of the discussion in this book the terms *disaster* and *mass casualty event* will be used interchangeably. But the basic distinction can be important and should be retained.

Mass casualty medicine consists in preparation for and provision of medical care or other health-preserving actions in mass casualty events or in situations where large numbers of casualties will result unless there is quick and decisive intervention. Considered thus, MCM combines clinical, public health, and public policy elements. The framework for ethical decision making employed in clinical mass casualty medicine—what I call the Rescue Paradigm (RP)—differs in important respects from the framework that operates in ordinary clinical medicine (OCM).

Health care in OCM centers on a dyadic relationship between clinician and patient. Clinicians see one patient at a time and endeavor to give each patient their full attention for the duration of the interchange. Generally, it is the patient who initiates contact, after experiencing symptoms or concerns that he or she interprets as medical problems. As the initiator, the patient retains a prerogative for framing the problem. That is to say, the patient's experience of illness usually begets and justifies the clinician's medical interventions. Nothing is a disease unless it can be related to experiences that patients generally find averse.[13] Clinicians may uncover data about latent processes and define these as diseases, but that is justified solely because such processes usually produce consequences that people dislike. In the end, it is up to the patient in any given clinical context to determine if an alleged disease is a medical problem that warrants specific interventions. A patient informed that he has mild seasonal allergic rhinitis, for instance, may decide that the symptoms (intermittent nasal congestion) evoked by this so-called malady are not significant and therefore not sufficiently worrisome to warrant further attention.

The notion that patients have ultimate authority to determine what counts as an intervention-worthy medical problem and to choose their interventions from an inventory of options offered and explained by the clinician is ensconced in bioethics' principle of autonomy. The ethical foundation for this principle resides for the most part in two facts and one ethical claim. The facts are (1) that different people have different and diverging notions of the "good" and the "right," and (2) that these diverging notions beget diverging operational concepts of health and illness, and diverging accounts of how to balance health against competing goods. The ethical claim is that each individual should have considerable latitude to interpret the concepts of "good" and "right," and hence also the concepts of "health" and "illness" as they apply to her own case.

Because they depend on contended values, the concepts of health and illness are hard to pin down. As objects of collective study or striving, they are frequently ambiguous, vague, and shifting. They are what I have called (following Charles Sanders Peirce) "dynamical objects"[14]—a term that underscores the way in which these incompletely differentiated concepts change as medical and social values evolve. It is in part this dynamic, indeterminate quality of health and illness that justifies bioethics' principle of autonomy.

In mass casualty medicine, many individuals simultaneously confront serious threats to health. Typically, few clinicians are properly situated to provide the needed medical care. With so many affected and so few there to help them, it is not possible to lavish the kind of time and attention on each patient that they would ordinarily receive. The clinical paradigm must change. Thus, ordinary clinical medicine (OCM), with its particular emphasis on the principle of autonomy, gives way to the Rescue Paradigm (RP)—named for its focus on snatching patients from the threat of death, dismemberment, and other dangers.

There is little time in RP for dynamical objects. Objectives, to the contrary, must be clear, solid, and relatively stationary. In distinction to OCM, the objects of striving in RP are rarely contended, debated, or even widely discussed. On most accounts, they are maximizing survival, minimizing serious morbidity, and (when possible) minimizing pain. The conjunction of these objects may be regarded as an "immediate object" for mass casualty medicine because it is well delineated, easily measurable, valued by virtually everyone, and widely assumed to be valued even by those who, in fact, do not value it highly. In RP, saving and preserving many is good; saving and preserving few is bad.

This conception of RP's immediate object is manifest in characterizations of the mission and ethics of disaster medicine. Emergency physician Eric Auf der Heide holds that clinicians serving in disasters should "do the greatest good for the greatest number of people." The U.S. Army's Soldier and Biological Chemical Command (SBCCOM) describes the mission in MCM as "providing the greatest benefit for the greatest number." Here "good" and "benefit" are not conceived in the usual vague utilitarian sense as "happiness," or even as good health. These authors are concerned with survival and the minimization of serious morbidity. Guidelines on triage, stabilization, transport, and disposition clearly reflect this preoccupation.

COERCION

With its intense focus on rescue and survival, the Rescue Paradigm begets a reciprocal de-emphasis on objectives such as the preservation of liberty, protection of property, and the cultivation of effective communal deliberation. In strategic formulations of the mission of RP, these objectives are frequently passed over without comment. Clinicians, for their part, have long been programmed to prioritize longevity and health over competing goods (a bias that bioethics sometimes purports to temper). The shift to RP allows clinicians to serve these causes in a more pristine, single-minded fashion.

A low threshold for coercion results when such single-mindedness combines with the widespread but misguided belief among clinicians and disaster planners that people are prone to extreme irrationality in mass casualty events.[15] In the tularemia scenario, Marcia Welby saves lives with aplomb, never considering that (1) her patient's apparently irrational decision might comport nicely with a divergent worldview that is as well justified in its own terms as Dr. Welby's is in hers; and (2) isolation or quarantine for "possibly contagious disease" may not be justified when used primarily to coerce a patient with a presumably noncontagious disease into accepting treatment. Whether Dr. Welby's decision was justified or not we shall examine later. For now, the point is that Welby dispenses with the usual dialogue, suspends patient decisional authority, and quickly resorts to coercion—all in service of RP and its imperative to save lives. In the remainder of the book, this sort of dynamic between coercion and values that drive mass casualty medicine will be a recurrent theme.

Beauchamp and Childress describe coercion as follows: "Coercion occurs if and only if one person intentionally uses a credible and severe threat of harm or force to control another."[16] This conception coheres fairly well with much of the more intricate, critical work on coercion by analytic philosophers such as Robert Nozick and Bernard Gert.[17] Coercion is differentiated from manipulation, which involves nonpersuasive psychological control exerted without threats of harm or force. However, there are a few qualifications that bear mention. First, the term "one person" (which reflects the interpersonal focus in much analytic ethics) is potentially misleading since, as Beauchamp and Childress illustrate in their discussion, coercion can be perpetrated by an institution such as a court or a public health agency. Second, for a threat of harm or force to be counted as coercion, it must exert some kind of influence on the persons who are objects of control. Merely *intending* to control others is not enough. Thus, Beauchamp and Childress write: "Whether coercion occurs depends on the subjective responses of the coercion's intended target."[18] Apparently they intend to capture this aspect of coercion with their use of the term "credible," though the primary import of credibility in my reading is that the threat will actually be carried out.

In light of these qualifications, coercion might be described as occurring if and only if *a person or group intentionally uses a credible and severe threat of harm or force to control others*, where "credible" is understood in the two senses described above. That is the conception that will pertain in this book. For the most part, we will be interested in threats of physical harm or physical force (i.e., threats that portend the possibility of violence). Some analysts might want to classify nonphysical threats of psychological harm or the use of psychological force as instances of coercion, but the fluctuant and imprecise boundaries of "psychological force" and "psychological harm" should make us cautious about casting too wide a net, especially given that these phenomena are covered in the notion of manipulation. Distinguishing threats of physical force and violence from purely psychological forms of manipulation is valuable, furthermore, in that it underscores the moral seriousness of physical force. Despite wide divergence among particular cultures and moralities on many ethical matters, diligent condemnation is directed almost universally toward unnecessary uses of physical force. This diligence is exhibited, for instance, in the ethical maxims offered by some thinkers as examples universal moral absolutes: "Do not kill an innocent person"; "Do not rape"; "Do not torture." These maxims may or may not be valid moral absolutes—but regardless, they are cited by moral absolutists just because they appeal to the universal revulsion for arbitrary violence. One could not generate the same impact, or the same level of agreement, with "Do not chastise the innocent" or "Do not offer irresistible enticements."

Coercion implies the infringement of liberty (though it is not the only way to infringe liberty).[19] Understood in the classical way, liberty signifies the absence of external impediments to action, "external" referring to sources outside the moral agent.[20] An "action," for our purposes, will consist of something that is intentionally and observably done. Ambulation, speech, thumb twiddling, and sipping porridge are examples. Sweating is not an action, because it is not done intentionally (though we may intentionally expose ourselves to conditions that cause sweating). Breathing and passing gas are usually not actions, but they can be when we focus on them (for instance, in practicing yoga or in attempting to make our 9-year-old laugh). Thinking is not an action in the public sense here denoted, since it is not observable (except by the thinker herself). However, it would be an action in a telepathic world.

Liberty is conceived in terms of the absence of external impediments. For our purposes, the only conceptual concern about these external impediments is how the threat of harm or force constitutes one—how coercion infringes liberty. Coercion infringes liberty in some circumstances by making certain actions impossible or (on some accounts) by creating reasons for not undertaking these actions that are so powerful that no rational person would disregard them. This type of coercion is infringement of liberty in the narrow sense (where perfect liberty requires only the absence of impediments that are essentially impervious).[21] Gert correlatively refers to this as the "narrow sense" of coercion. Sometimes, however, coercion infringes liberty only in the sense that threats of harm or force act as deterrents that most people in the target population will find dissuasive. This type of coercion infringes liberty in the wide sense (where liberty requires the absence of all serious impediments, even potentially pervious ones). Accordingly, Gert identifies such instances of coercion as examples of the "wide sense" of coercion.[22] In what follows, we will regard coercion as including both narrow and wide senses (and thus liberty also as including both narrow and wide senses).

Not everything that is heinous is coercion. And not all coercion is heinous. The category of heinous-things-not-coercive includes, for example, illicit enticements such as researchers offering inordinate sums of money to lower-income subjects for participating in dangerous, poorly designed experiments. This is not coercion because no threat of harm or force is introduced by the manipulating party. In the category of coercive-things-not-heinous we would include speed limits and income taxes (though I suppose some citizens do regard these as heinous). These are coercive because they are backed by credible threats of force.

Because the term *coercion* resonates with moral overtones, many attempts to co-opt and refashion it have occurred over history as various ideologues try to gain the moral high ground. Interestingly, Gaylin and Jennings recognize that "the term *coercion* has been extended to include almost every conceivable external influence on behavior."[23] Yet rather than sticking with the more restricted sense of coercion predominant in the natural language, these authors impart their own batch of idiosyncrasies. Though they admit that physical force "is the prototypical case of coercion," they claim without explanation that coercion really is not physical at all, and opine (defying the widespread notion of "psychological constraints") that only "constraint" is fundamentally physical in nature. In this vein they write: "One reason for separating constraint from coercion is that whereas constraint can well be physical, for all practical purposes coercion cannot be. The generalized misconception of coercion as involving physical force must be laid to rest. Coercion must be perceived as the psychological phenomenon it inevitably is."[24]

The linguistic essentialism in this passage is startling. Gaylin and Jennings focus on psychological similarities between reward-motivating and harm-avoidance-motivating interactions, then isolate these as the single, deep meaning of "coercion" — missed over the ages even by those who initially coined the term. Now they will set things aright.[25]

Beauchamp and Childress, on the other hand, elaborate a concept of coercion that reflects longstanding everyday usage (not to mention Latin roots). It is hard to imagine what sort of argument Gaylin and Jennings might bring against them (neither party addresses the other in the cited texts), except to point out that their (i.e., Gaylin and Jennings's) newfangled conception of coercion has caught on with some bioethicists (especially those working in research ethics), to assert their moral authority to construct and canonize a new semantics and to conclude that when lay persons, intellectuals, and other bioethicists fail to recognize the new canon, they are suffering from a "generalized misconception." But that is a bad argument.

In any case, we will stick with the ordinary conception of coercion articulated by Beauchamp and Childress. Readers who prefer the Gaylin and Jennings version can nevertheless take heart, since the crucial cases and practices considered in what follows would be classified as coercive on either scale. Some readers may also be uncomfortable with the notion of "liberty" here elaborated, since arguably it precludes some of the species of "positive liberty" that are currently being elaborated. For our purposes, however, differences about the definition of liberty are even less concerning than differences about coercion, since our focus on negative liberties merely reflects an empirical reality — that these are the types of liberty that are most directly and seriously impinged when quarantine, conscription, mandatory treatment, and other measures considered in this book are enacted. No effort will be made to dissuade those who insist on the existence of positive liberties or the moral right of citizens to have these fulfilled.

THE MODEL STATE EMERGENCY HEALTH POWERS ACT

Even before September 11, 2001, the Clinton and Bush administrations worried about disaster preparations. As TopOff and other exercises seemed to demonstrate,[26] state laws governing emergency quarantine, property acquisition, and other coercive measures were frequently incomplete, incongruent, and confusing or ambiguous; they were poorly coordinated with the laws of bordering states and largely inadequate to cover the exigencies of bioterrorism and other contemporary threats.[27] Many state laws had not been closely examined or revised for fifty or more years, often surviving unmodified from the days of yellow fever, cholera, and smallpox in the eighteenth and nineteenth centuries. With these pitfalls in mind, the Centers for Disease Control (CDC) commissioned legal and public health scholars to produce model legislation that states could consider when updating their emergency preparedness statutes.[28] In collaboration with organizations representing national and state policy makers and public health officials,[29] these scholars produced the Model State Emergency Health Powers Act (MSEHPA), the initial draft of which was released for public commentary on October 23, 2001. After numerous criticisms were considered and amendments made,[30] another draft appeared on December 21, 2001.[31] Many states responded by enacting statutes that incorporated facets of the model act.[32]

MSEHPA contains provisions for many of the coercive interventions that are likely in forensic disasters or other mass casualty events. According to MSEHPA, some of these provisions should pertain under ordinary circumstances, prior to a public health emergency. Mandatory reporting (within 24 hours) of any condition that may be a potential cause of a public health emergency applies at all times in MSEHPA to health care providers, coroners, medical examiners, pharmacists, veterinarians, persons owning livestock or caring for animals, and laboratories (Section 301). Public health officials are also granted routine authority, "for examination purposes," to "close, evacuate, or decontaminate any facility or decontaminate or destroy any material when the authority reasonably suspects that such facility or material may endanger the public health" (Section 302(c)).[33]

Other provisions of MSEHPA go into effect only after the governor has declared a public health emergency. In such circumstances, the public health authority is granted power to take control of or condemn facilities, including health care facilities, and to regulate all forms of transportation. It is also empowered to require health care facilities and businesses, by threat of force, to provide particular services. All materials (especially health care supplies, communication devices, fuels, food, and clothing) are susceptible to inspection, rationing, seizure, decontamination, and commerce restrictions (Sections 502, 503, and 505). Public health workers can take possession or control of human remains and take facilities and resources to store or dispose of them (Section 504). However, just compensation is to be provided by the government for facilities and materials that are taken or destroyed, except when the action was taken because the facilities and materials were believed to endanger the public's health (Sections 506 and 507). During a public health emergency, citizens can be required to submit to medical examinations, tests, vaccinations, or treatment and subjected to isolation or quarantine if they refuse (Sections 602 and 603). When necessary (i.e., when less restrictive means are not adequate) any individual or group may be isolated or quarantined at home or at other private and public premises—with provisions made for medical observation, treatment, and adequate food, clothing, shelter, and communication (Section 604).[34] As a condition of licensure or the privilege to practice, the public health authority can require in-state health care providers to assist in whichever medical activities it deems necessary (Section 608). Broad immunity is granted to the state and its officials, and to organizations and persons cooperating with them, except for gross negligence or willful misconduct (Section 804).

By putting together a formal proposal and offering it to the public for scrutiny, the authors of MSEHPA have helped to initiate public dialogue about the legitimate uses of coercion in MCM. They offer both an inventory of likely forms of coercion and a legal framework to guide their implementation. With respect to the former, it is important to know that their inventory is not complete (nor does it claim to be). Coercive acts are also likely to occur, for example, as police secure the boundaries of a hot zone at the site of a chemical attack, or when rescuers triage victims. They occur when speech is restricted in order to prevent a mass casualty event (e.g., in preventing the publication of research that terrorists might use)[35] and in routine market restrictions (e.g., in preventing pharmaceutical companies from manufacturing smallpox immunizations for sale to the public). With respect to the legal framework, there is already much contention.

The Preamble to MSEHPA begins with the now customary reference to the September 11 attacks, followed by a statement that "our nation realizes that the government's foremost responsibility is to protect the health, safety, and well being of its citizens." Contrary to this claim, many American citizens believe that protecting citizens' rights, including civil liberties, stands alongside security as the government's foremost responsibility—and that a mandate to protect well-being is potentially dangerous because it is too open-ended. Predictably, these parties reacted negatively to MSEHPA.

George Annas led the assault with an article in the *New England Journal of Medicine* that identified the following major problems with MSEHPA: (1) "It is not clear what problem the model act is intended to solve" (Annas does not accept that the stated problem is really a problem); (2) the act provides public health authority that is too broad; (3) putting public health authorities in charge of a bioterrorist attack does not always make sense; (4) "there is no evidence" that health care providers or citizens will be reluctant to cooperate with legitimate public health interventions; and (5) even if quarantine laws were needed, they should be federal laws, not state laws.[36] At the crux of Annas's argument is the fear that coercive public health measures will undermine public trust, resulting in less compliance and a less satisfactory response to bioterrorism events than we could expect if officials respected civil rights and worked hand in hand with the public. "Provisions that treat citizens as the enemy, with the use of the police for enforcement," Annas writes, "are much more likely to cost lives than to save them."[37]

Yet paradoxically, some supporters of MSEHPA argue that a fundamental reason for adopting coercive public health laws is that they will *enhance* solidarity and trust.[38]

TRUST

Mark Hall describes three stances regarding trust in health care. His focus is on the trust that patients and the public manifest for clinicians and other persons involved in the provision of health care.[39] For the *predicated* stance, the existence of trust is assumed, and attempts are made to ensure that clinicians live up to this trust. For the *supportive* stance, trust is regarded as fragile but important, so efforts are made to cultivate it. Finally, for the *substitutive* stance,[40] trust is regarded as absent or unwarranted, such that third-party oversight and regulation are necessary as substitutes.

These approaches also operate in mass casualty medicine, but here the loci and dynamics of trust are somewhat different. As with ordinary clinical medicine, there are relations of trust (or mistrust) between patients and clinicians. Of similar or perhaps even greater importance, however, is trust (or mistrust) manifested by the public for government officials, public health authorities, and other parties primarily responsible for overseeing operations in MCM. Finally, the issue of how much authorities and clinicians trust the public is critical in MCM (it is arguably also critical yet neglected in OCM).

In the dialogue about MSEHPA, focus is placed on the second species of trust (i.e., public trust for the authorities). As implied above, a supportive approach is employed on both sides of the debate. One party thinks we should support public trust by upholding a commitment to civil rights; the other party thinks that trust is enhanced by evidence of preparedness—including provisions for necessary forms of coercion. Interestingly, both Gostin and Annas foresee occasions in which it is necessary to adopt a substitutive approach. However, they have different perceptions of when and how this necessity is likely to arise, which leads them to recommend different forms of substitution. Gostin and his colleagues worry that an absence or paucity of trust will beget low levels of cooperation. Hence, they foresee a need to introduce coercive measures as the substitute. Annas and his cohorts are not as concerned about a paucity of trust as they are that trust may not be warranted. The prerogative to institute coercive measures such as quarantines and takings (property expropriations), on this view, is about the worst thing that could happen in such a situation, since it places greater power in the hands of the parties who do not warrant trust. When trust is not warranted, the substitute must consist in measures to hold authorities accountable. A strict adherence to civil rights—including a willingness to punish public officials who violate them—is Annas's preferred strategy.

In sum, both Gostin and Annas want to establish conditions in which health officials responsible for overseeing MCM are highly trustworthy and also deeply trusted. Both worry, however, about mistrust. Gostin seems to believe that mistrust is endemic and almost inevitable in public health emergencies, despite the general trustworthiness of authorities. Annas believes that levels of trust are generally adequate and tend to surge in public health emergencies, but he fears that untrustworthy health officials will undermine it. With respect to MSEHPA, Gostin thinks it provides a necessary substitute when trust is insufficient while also enhancing trust so that coercive measures become less likely. Annas believes that MSEHPA damages trust and that it is unnecessary and wrongly conceived.

The enormously complex permutations of trust and its causal interdependence with factors such as justification, legitimacy, ideology, power, authority, cooperation, and innovation constitute a major challenge for anyone hoping to flesh out an ethical framework for public health interventions. Our project on coercion in mass casualty medicine is especially burdened by this challenge because it requires not merely a general ethical framework but also a reckoning on how things change in times of unspeakable tragedy. As a preface, we will consider recent attempts at constructing a general framework for public health ethics.

CHAPTER TWO

Public Health and Its Ethical Basis

According to the Institute of Medicine (IOM), "Public health is what we, as a society, do collectively to assure the conditions for people to be healthy."[1] Using the systems terminology so popular (though imprecisely understood) in health care commentary, we might rephrase this definition: "Public health is a social subsystem ordered around the stabilization and enhancement of parameters that signify the existence of conditions for people to be healthy."

Several factors related to this conception of public health bear mention. First, as I have observed, the conditions for good health are often established through coercion. This chapter will investigate general approaches to justifying coercive measures in public health. Second, conditions for good health are not equivalent to good health itself, and some thinkers believe that the latter is actually the primary aim of public health. Hence, rather than targeting parameters that signify conditions for people to be healthy (e.g., clean air and clean water), as the IOM definition suggests, public health authorities often target parameters that signify the presence of good health (e.g., long life span, low morbidity rates). For individuals who understand public health in the latter way, the conditions for good health are not enough; these individuals are satisfied only when people are taking advantage of such conditions so as to live healthy lives. The practical consequence of this latter view is public health practice ordered around the stabilization and enhancement of parameters that signify good health. Third, the concept of health is subservient to, and ordered around, the conception of a "good life." Because various people and moral communities disagree about the good life, they also disagree about the meaning of health and about its importance as a constituent of the good life. This implies that the concept of health will be elusive and value-laden and that the need for particular public health measures will be disputed. People who conceive the good life as active and athletic, for instance, will have a higher estimate of the level of physical endurance and muscular strength that is required for "good health" than sedentary people will.[2] The former group might be more supportive of health interventions that promote exercise (e.g., public construction of bicycle paths).

INDIVIDUAL RIGHTS VERSUS THE COMMON GOOD

Because threats of force are ethically significant and usually avoided where possible, a general willingness to use them for the promotion of health signifies that — despite differing opinions about its meaning and significance — most people value health highly. I take that as an indisputable empirical verity. At the same time, however, people value other things besides health. The authors of America's Declaration of Independence, for instance, identified rights to "life, liberty, and the pursuit of happiness" as politically fundamental human goods. None of these good things is synonymous with good health, though "life" implies, at a minimum, a beating heart, and "the pursuit of happiness" would presumably be very difficult for someone in especially poor health.

The (disputed) inventory of human goods contains certain elements that potentially conflict with good health. It is therefore common for public health analysts to recognize the need for a "proper balance" between good health (which they typically describe with population-based parameters) and other goods with which it may be in tension. Often this tension is described in terms of a polarity between "individual interests" (or "individual rights") and "the common good" — as if these entities were two differing and frequently opposed species of human good. In this vein, Amitai Etzioni characterizes the challenge of public health in an age of bioterrorism as managing the "difficult balance between individual rights and the common good."[3] Given the recently heightened public awareness of terrorist threats, emerging infectious diseases, and so forth, Etzioni and others have issued calls to reassess the proper proportion between these two apparently countervailing values. Lawrence Gostin, primary author of MSEHPA, writes: "The balance between individual interests and common goods needs to be recalibrated in an age of terrorism."[4]

The alleged tension between individual interests and the common good parallels the struggle between "individualism" and "communitarianism" that dominated political philosophy throughout much of the 1980s and 90s in that it hinges on a community-centered or aggregate notion of the "common good" pitted against individual values, rights, or interests. To clarify, it is helpful to consider some of the prominent accounts of the meaning of "common good."

PUBLIC HEALTH AND THE COMMON GOOD

Just as competing conceptions of the office of public health hinge on opinions about whether the task of public health is to establish the conditions for good health or to establish good health itself, competing conceptions of the common good hinge on opinions about whether the polis should establish the *conditions* for living good lives (e.g., liberty to pursue material wealth, protection from violence, and conditions for good health) or establish the *elements* of good lives (e.g., material possessions, cultural enrichments, and good health). Those who think the polis is tasked with establishing the conditions for living well tend to conceive the common good in terms of parameters designed to signify such conditions (e.g., indices of economic freedom or civil liberty, crime statistics, and immunization rates). We will call these versions of the common good "conditions models." Those, on the other hand, who think the polis is tasked with establishing the elements of good lives tend to conceive the common good in terms of parameters that express whether or not people are actually living good lives (e.g., poverty rates, indices of equality between disparate cultural groups, and morbidity rates). We'll call these versions "fulfillment models."

The distinction between conditions and fulfillments is not hard-and-fast, since any experience of conditions for good living will beget a sense of living well and hence will to a degree comprise one of the elements of a good life. Conversely, most of what we would identify as elements of good living—for example, material possessions and good health—exhibit instrumental qualities that help beget other fulfillments. In this sense, most of the elements of a good life are also conditions for living better, just as most of the conditions for a good life are fulfillments that constitute part of a good life. Nevertheless, a distinction between conditions and fulfillments stands, in a rough but important qualitative sense, on a difference in degree. Some goods are primarily instrumental; others are valued primarily for their intrinsic properties.

The distinction is further muddied by the tendency of those within the first group (conditions supporters) to defend their approach by arguing that promoting conditions for good living is a better means for establishing the elements of good lives than is targeting these elements directly.[5] Likewise, some members of the other group (fulfillments supporters) focus on the instrumental qualities of their favored fulfillments, and characterize themselves merely as proponents of a more robust conditions account. This bilateral appeal to fulfillments is important not only in that it provides common ground for debate between the diverging parties but also in the sense that it expresses commonality at a fundamental theoretical level—that is, both parties tend to believe (though there are a few dissenters) that living well is the ultimate justification for the polis. Disagreement hinges on opinions about how explicit and direct the state's role should be in defining and cultivating such good lives.

Fulfillment models of the common good come in three important varieties: utilitarian, egalitarian, and broadly communitarian. *Utilitarians* measure fulfillments in the aggregate, without specific regard to discrepancies between value-experiencing agents (i.e., persons). For instance, some utilitarians hold that happiness is the good and hence conceive the common good as a state of maximal overall happiness.[6] They are willing to tolerate the existence of numerous wretchedly miserable persons— even if these persons have done nothing in particular to warrant such wretchedness— so long as the aggregate happiness is served (many utilitarians hold, however, that the possibility of arbitrary wretchedness undermines everyone's happiness).

Egalitarians also frequently employ aggregate measurements, but they impose an important side-constraint on the utilitarian calculus: fulfillment—or at least some minimal level of fulfillment—must, as far as human powers permit, be universal. Hence, egalitarians insist that we cannot sacrifice specific individuals or groups on behalf of aggregate fulfillment. They tend to conceive the common good as maximal overall fulfillment, given the egalitarian side-constraint.[7]

Broadly *communitarian* conceptions of the common good focus on the cultivation of fulfillments that embody the shared memories and expectations of moral communities.[8] On this view, solidarity and a common cultural heritage are often normatively pivotal considerations. Some communitarian thinkers, however, believe that pluralistic jurisdictions such as the United States have too few common values and ideals to justify a robust, broadly communitarian political conception of the common good. Such thinkers usually choose a conditions model of the common good when formulating political strategies, focusing on the maintenance of conditions that facilitate the emergence of viable and relatively self-sufficient natural communities.[9]

Conditions models of the common good are, in fact, supported by a wide variety of theorists who tend to share a common conviction that conceptions of the good life vary too immensely among individuals and groups in pluralistic nations like the United States to justify a particular state-sponsored conception of the good life. Sometimes the endorsement of a conditions model is very tentative and amounts in practice to a fulfillment model. John Rawls, for instance, defines the common good as "certain general conditions that are in an appropriate sense equally to everyone's advantage."[10] These conditions, it turns out, include several "primary goods"[11] distributed in accordance with a Rawlsian formulation of the egalitarian side-constraint. In order to establish what should count as a primary good, and how these goods should be ranked in relation to other goods, Rawls employs a fairly robust conception of the good life. Though he refers to this conception as a "thin theory" of the good, subsequent analysis (not only by critics, but by Rawls himself) has shown that his thin theory is too thick to garner the kind of wide, overlapping consensus that he desires.[12] In the end, his conception of the common good stretches well beyond the minimalism of the conditions model.

In addition to fulfillment models and conditions models of the common good, there is what Alex John London calls the "corporate conception," in which the common good is identified with community interests that are "distinct from those of its individual members."[13] The first salient property (not acknowledged by London) of the corporate conception is that virtually no one explicitly endorses it. It cannot be identified with communitarianism, since most communitarians do not divorce the interests of the community from the interests of its members. Even America's grand old philosopher of community, Josiah Royce, who holds that communities are higher-order persons, identifies the interests of communities with the deepest interests of the human individuals who embody and serve them.[14] The second salient property of this conception (also not acknowledged by London) is that it frequently operates as a kind of subliminal default for persons disaffected by selfish indulgences that sometimes accompany individualism and the exercise of individual rights. In this mindset, it is easy enough (so long as one refrains from detailed analysis) to conjure the feeling that collective values are distinct from and superior to the ends pursued by individuals. As such a subliminal ideal, the corporate conception is important. The third salient property of this conception (highlighted by London) is its all-or-nothing triggering mechanism as a rationale for infringing individual rights. "Given the corporate conception of the common good," London writes, "something poses a threat to the common good—meets the triggering condition—only if it jeopardizes the continued existence or proper functioning of society as a whole. . . . Notice, however, that once something *is* deemed to threaten the common good, the corporate conception yields only the weakest possible practical constraint on what can be done in response."[15] Disasters and terrorist threats are examples of potent triggering mechanisms.

The corporate conception of the common good is presumed by anyone who refers to a fundamental conflict between individual interests and the common good (since it is not possible to conceive of ongoing conflict between individual interests and collective interests unless one regards these interests as substantially distinct).

The increased frequency of such references during our current "war on terrorism" is consistent with London's conception of the triggering condition. At the same time, lack of explicit endorsements for the corporate conception—even by eminent scholars who seem to presume it—is also striking. Gostin, for instance, writes at length about the tension between "individual interests" (or, in some formulations, "individual rights") and "common goods," yet never offers a detailed description of the common good.[16]

For proponents of the conditions model or the fulfillment model of the common good, the notion of conflict between individual interests and the common good is incoherent, since the common good is conceived, on both models, as a system of individual interests or rights. Unsurprisingly,[17] London lumps the two models together in what he calls the "generic interests conception"[18] and contrasts this conception with the corporate conception.

The upshot of this characterization of conceptions of the common good is that describing the ethical challenge of public health interventions as a balancing act between individual interests and the common good is untenable. For most thinkers, the common good is constituted by a subset of individual interests. Hence, tension between individual interests and the common good amounts to tension between one group of individual interests and another group of individual interests. Focus on the tension between individual *rights* and the common good fares only a little better. Our formulation of the fulfillment model admits this form of tension so long as the notion of rights is tightly restricted—for instance, by including only negative rights (classic liberties)[19] or civil liberties. Ultimately, however, this view would be unsatisfactory for proponents of both the conditions and the fulfillment models of the common good, since: (1) on conditions models, the common good is promoted largely by cultivating an environment where negative rights and civil liberties are protected and the common good is thus coextensive with the realm of negative and civil rights; and (2) virtually all current versions of the fulfillment model insist on the provision of positive rights.

Perhaps, then, there are better ways of formulating the ethical challenge of justifying intrusive public health interventions, including coercive ones.

PUBLIC HEALTH AND SECURITY

In a previous essay, I suggested that certain medical and public health interventions (including government-sponsored access to a basic minimum of health care) should be regarded as matters of national security.[20] Now I want to buttress that argument with another contention: *The primary ethical challenge confronting any ini-*

tiative for intrusive public health measures is the difficulty of properly balancing security needs and liberties. Public health, as we noted, is concerned with the stabilization and enhancement of parameters that signify the existence of conditions for people to be healthy. These parameters are properly regarded as proxies or indices of collective security from illness and injury. They are closely related to (and at times overlap with) parameters that characterize law enforcement and military objectives—the latter being involved with collective security from physical intrusions, aggression, and violence. Intrusive public health and law enforcement measures nearly always infringe liberties, including state-protected liberties (parameters stabilized and enhanced by the political system) such as freedom of movement, freedom of association, control of private property, and so forth. In other words, the tension between security needs and liberties is a ubiquitous factor in public health and law enforcement.

One key consideration in achieving a proper balance between securities and liberties is the realization that public health agencies, law enforcement agencies, and other social units that can threaten liberties are subsystems of the larger polis. When the architects and agents of such subsystems begin to regard their organizations as stand-alone systems with tasks unqualified by higher-order mandates, ethical problems ensue. This posture is typified in public health by the World Health Organization (WHO).

The first director of WHO, Dr. Brock Chisholm, advised the world that the task of international public health was unbounded and unqualified: "The world is sick and the ills are due to the perversion of man: his inability to live with himself. The microbe is not the enemy: science is sufficiently advanced to cope with it were it not for the barriers of superstition. . . . [Hence] the scope of the task before the committee knows no bounds."[21] In line with this view, WHO defines health as "a state of complete physical, mental, and social well-being and not merely the absence of disease or infirmity."[22] In other words, WHO believes that health is *the* comprehensive human good and that WHO is its appointed guardian. Currently, many people turn to priests, family elders, and moral communities for guidance about the meaning and pursuit of well-being. But for Chisholm, these habits are manifestations of superstition—barriers that need to be eradicated. In the enlightened future, people will consult physicians and public health authorities. Substantial forms of moral pluralism—those based on differences of opinion about the meaning of "well-being"—will be a thing of the past.

This posture is ethically problematic because it preempts the strife of ideas between parties that harbor diverging conceptions of the right and the good. Chisholm does not derail their arguments or prove them wrong; he merely asserts the authority of his own secular humanistic view. To overcome his adversaries, he would need to garner and deploy great dollops of political, police, and military power. And that, indeed, sometimes seems to be the strategy of WHO.

So far, the megalomania of WHO founders has not taken hold in the United States (or elsewhere, though it seems to be more viable in secular humanistic Western Europe). In the United States, health is regarded as only one aspect of human flourishing, and proposals for intrusive public health measures need to be justified in relation to other conditions or aspects of the common good. On the other hand, public health workers and public policy makers in the United States are not immune from moral imperialism. Sometimes the justification for coercive public health interventions that tread on others' conceptions of the good life amounts to little more than glib assertion of policy makers' moral visions. I was introduced to this occurrence (and my own complicity) several years ago by a relative from my wife's side of the family—Uncle Rocky. His story may be instructive.

Uncle Rocky is a Harley Davidson enthusiast who has spent much of his life riding with a rough-hewn biker crowd. At a family reunion, Rocky asked about my work as an emergency physician and my experience as a mountaineer. He wanted me to explain why emergency physicians go to such length to promote legislation that coerces bikers into using motorcycle helmets, while essentially ignoring things like mountaineering safety (for instance, we could save lives by promoting legislation that requires mountaineers to wear helmets). After all, he observed, mountaineering seems as dangerous as biking. I responded that it is not simply a matter of dangerousness. Mountaineering accidents are not the public health problem that motorcycle accidents are, since fewer people climb than ride motorcycles. If the number of people dying while climbing started to approach the number dying on motorcycles, I continued, mountaineering safety legislation would surely follow.

Rocky didn't accept this explanation. If saving large numbers of lives was really a sufficient reason for public health legislation, he observed, then we wouldn't stop at saving a few hundred lives with motorcycle helmet laws; we'd go ahead and save tens of thousands by cutting traffic speed limits down to about 25 miles per hour. Ultimately, I was forced to concede that attempts to justify public health legislation on the basis either of reducing dangerousness or of reducing total numbers of fatalities were not applied uniformly to all public health threats. I conceded that there is little chance that we will cut the speed limits to 25 miles per hour, regardless of the weight of evidence that might demonstrate the public health effectiveness of such a measure. Policy makers, like most of the rest of us, like to drive fast. Forcing everyone to crawl along at 25 miles per hour would significantly impinge on everyone's quality of life.

And this is where Uncle Rocky seized the moment. From his vantage point, Nirvana consists in hugging the seat of his Harley as the wind whistles through his (now mostly absent) hair. That is the good life. "Who," he asked and I paraphrase, "is the government to tell me that I have no right to live my own life as I see fit? If I am hurt or I die on my bike, then I am a lucky man who has died in the saddle. I'm insured, and I pay my own funeral or medical expenses. Yet with the helmet laws, if I fail to pay the tickets, additional fines are added. If I refuse to pay the fines, they'll try to take me to jail. And when they come to haul me away, I'll fight back—probably losing in a bloody way. Uncle Sam, in order to keep me safe, is willing to kill me. Does that make sense?"

Rocky's point is worth reflection. When safety legislation is backed by the police power, violence and physical harm are its ultimate sanctions. This correlation should induce caution in the use of coercion to prevent self-harm. Now contrast Uncle Rocky's lifelong pursuit of wind-in-the-hair and his wariness about government paternalism with the orientation of public health ethicist Dan Beauchamp, who writes: "The fear of democratic government—especially the American democratic government—as the national nanny is, in the end, rather silly."[23] Ultimately, that is the only rejoinder that public health has for Uncle Rocky. His view of the good life, and his uneasiness about the police power, are just silly.

To his credit, Beauchamp (who remains silent about motorcycle helmets in the above-cited book) distinguishes between public health legislation that is legitimate and that which reflects unreasonable "moralism." He illustrates legitimate interventions by alluding, for example, to seatbelt laws. There is no moralism here, I think most would agree, just a recognition that many people are relatively unconscious of the risk they take by not using seatbelts and that people with the bad habit of not buckling up will live better lives—even by their own personal standards—if they are jostled out of the bad habits with seatbelt laws. No one (or hardly anyone) fails to buckle up because they think the good life requires driving without a seatbelt.

As for moralism, it is hard to sort out Beauchamp's view. In some cases he approves of moralism as a public health tool—as in propaganda to induce disapproval of smoking and excessive drinking. On the other hand, he seems to be strongly repulsed by disapproval of sexual promiscuity and by other forms of disapproval that he personally finds overwrought or "extreme." How he would feel about disapproval directed to bikers' lifestyles is anyone's guess, but the reader gets the feeling that Beauchamp is very comfortable using his own moral compass to guide public policy. That sort of comfort among policy-making elites makes people like Rocky uncomfortable—and distrustful. Despite a profusion of rhetoric about collective goods, solidarity, and community, Beauchamp offers no formula for a proper balance between security and liberty. He merely presumes that his sense of the matter is better (for everyone) than Uncle Rocky's, or Theodore Roosevelt's, or the equilibrium that would be recommended by any number of other high-adrenaline personalities who think that danger enhances the quality of living.

Uncle Rocky's argument hinges on the assumption that riding motorcycles without a helmet is self-threatening but does not harm others in a significant way. Should Rocky's non-helmet-use present others with responsibilities to provide or fund his medical care, his argument would be threatened (though presumably bikers could be required to carry insurance).[24] But we would have to show that the harm to others is substantial enough to warrant our threat of violence against Rocky. Though no potentially dangerous actions are purely self-regarding as to their harms, it is clear that in some instances the threatened harms are largely self-regarding. Just as clearly, riding a motorcycle without a helmet is one of these cases.

The prevention of self-harm (PSH) is one of three general rationales that found public health interventions, and it is clearly the most controversial. Examples of the PSH rationale in mass casualty medicine include proposals to ban persons from obtaining immunization against smallpox and mandatory decontamination of victims at the site of chemical spills or attacks (though PSH is not the primary rationale in cases where decontamination is needed to prevent contaminated individuals from harming others). PSH is least controversial when it is applied to legally incompetent persons (e.g., in the prevention of childhood accidents). As we will discuss in a subsequent chapter, there may be reason for presuming that large-scale public incompetence will pertain for particular exigent decisions that need to be made in mass casualty events. That would open the door for PSH.

Coercion is more frequently (and less controversially) justified as a measure to prevent individuals from harming other parties. Let us call this rationale PHO (preventing harm to others). PHO applies in coercive measures like isolation and quarantine, roadway speed limits, immunization laws, directly observed treatment programs, and industrial emissions standards. A third rationale for coercion is to garner resources that are needed to enhance the health of others (EHO). This justification applies in takings (such as the appropriation of private property for an improvised hospital) and in the conscription of health care workers during public health emergencies.

PRETHEORETICAL APPROACHES TO THE ETHICS OF COERCION
IN PUBLIC HEALTH

Before proceeding (in the next chapter) with detailed arguments for the justification of coercion in public health and mass casualty medicine, I should acknowledge that the need for ethical arguments is not always recognized in public health practice. There are, in fact, three major pretheoretical approaches to the use of coercion in public health, and only one of them acknowledges the relevance of ethical arguments.

The first approach has been called the "positivist" approach.[25] According to positivists, public health is a scientific discipline unconcerned with values and ethics. On this model, society decides that it wants to pursue certain health-related objectives, and public health scientists supply the facts about how this can be accomplished. Facts and values, then, are clearly distinguished—the former being the business of scientists, the latter falling to society. Formally speaking, positivism can be defined as the claim that (1) human knowledge pertains only to testable, objective, causal relations, and hence that (2) a hypothesis or statement is epistemically meaningful if and only if it is possible (at least in theory) to test it with experiments that directly verify or falsify it, or directly show that its strict implications do or do not pertain.

A particularly difficult problem for public health positivists is that their primary object of study—health—is a value-laden concept. If meaningful statements must be empirically testable, how are we to construct a meaningful statement that defines health? The concept of good health evolves only from the experience of suffering and illness (health being the freedom from such things).[26] But suffering is subjective, and the meaning of illness also seems to reside largely in the visors of the afflicted.[27]

For instance, we conceive of hyperlipidemia (high cholesterol and fat levels in the blood) as a disease. It is a disease because it leads to events such as myocardial infarction (MI) and stroke that most people perceive as afflictions. If it didn't lead to such events, it would be classified as a normal variant (and a very common one). Now the judgment that MI and stroke are afflictions, and thus bad things, leads to judgments that they are illnesses or manifestations of disease. That is a value judgment. Apart from such valuation, there is no "scientific" way to establish that MI and stroke are manifestations of disease, and hence also no way of showing that hyperlipidemia is a disease. One could argue that they are normal human processes that help in keeping the population young and dynamic. But such an argument does not reflect the socially dominant moral visions of human flourishing and the human life cycle. So on the basis of a collective moral vision, we classify hyperlipidemia, MI, and stroke as health problems.

"Normal function," as so many commentators have observed, is never value-free.[28] Even when it is conceived as a statistical regularity, its boundaries are arbitrary and its status is normatively obscure. Positivists seem to want to say that certain variations from normal are bad—for example, ones that lead to short life spans and suffering—and that others are not. But this approach makes sense only if we endorse the hypothesis that shorter lives and miserable lives are negative things that ought to be avoided (rather than merely things that many people arbitrarily condemn). Unfortunately for the positivists, that hypothesis is not empirically testable in the manner they prescribe. As a final nail in the positivist coffin, it turns out that affirmations of positivism are themselves not testable; so if positivism is true, it is by its own tenets scientifically meaningless. Unsurprisingly, positivism was abandoned long ago by most philosophers of science.

A second approach—now probably the dominant one—to the justification of coercion in public health is based on ethical dogmatism. In this version, the existence of value-driven public health practice is acknowledged, but ethical arguments are eschewed because theorists are confident that they already understand the salient values. Concepts like "health" and "social justice" are regarded as obvious and fixed. Public health workers of this ilk frequently view themselves as "advocates" for social justice or a healthier public.

Social justice advocacy in public health is remarkable insofar as there is probably no single ethical concept that elicits such a divergence of opinion and such contentious debate among educated persons as the concept of justice. Yet in the scholarly public health literature, this contentiousness is typically ignored and the terms "justice" and "social justice" bandied about as if their meanings were uncontroversial and fixed.[29] For proponents of the dogmatic approach, it is as if the ideas of Locke, Madison, Mill, Nozick, and Hayek were never expressed.

The dogmatist approach is more difficult to defeat than the positivist approach because it is so unreflective. Positivists offer arguments, and these can be challenged by counterarguments. But how does one deal with an assertion put forth by someone who is not interested in hearing or addressing counterassertions? The only answer, I believe, is to keep pressing the challenge. That is part of the mission of this book.

In summary, the positivist version views public health as a domain of facts only and leaves the values to society. The dogmatist version acknowledges that public health involves both facts and values but thinks that the values are well-established.

Neither has any use for serious ethical arguments or inquiry. This book assumes a third approach, one that views public health practice as a domain of both facts and values, and considers both facts and values to be legitimate objects of inquiry. I will call this the pluralist approach because it acknowledges the plurality of moral visions and our need to mediate them through a process of deliberation, discussion, and inquiry.

CHAPTER THREE

Legitimacy

Five years into the First World War, sailors and soldiers started dying en masse in Boston and at Fort Devens, Massachusetts. Initially, the Germans were blamed, since—so the thinking went—if Germans introduced lethal chemicals such as chlorine and phosgene gas into battlefields, they were capable of seeding cities with killer microbes.[1] Now they had imported a killer virus in Bayer aspirin bottles. Or perhaps they snuck the pathogens in by sea—commandos swimming ashore with vials of microorganisms for dispersion in theaters and at war rallies.[2]

But it wasn't the Germans. And the epidemic wasn't confined to America's eastern seaboard. It was part of the worldwide reemergence of an influenza strain—"Spanish flu"—that had run a much milder course the preceding spring. In the fall it got vicious. Unlike ordinary flu, this bug sought out the young and vigorous. Men and women slid in a matter of hours from normalcy to critical illness: burning with fever, gasping for air, coughing blood—and struggling for comprehension. Schools closed to become makeshift morgues. In the worst-hit areas, bodies were stacked like cordwood.

In a few months, influenza killed more Americans than heart disease, cancer, strokes, diabetes, emphysema, AIDS, and Alzheimer disease combined now kill in a year.[3] Overall, it was the worst human loss of life from any disease over a similar duration in the recorded history of the world,[4] killing far more than the combat dead in World War I or even in World War II. In the United States, life expectancy changed in one year as a result of this epidemic, from 51 years to 39 years.[5]

The public health response to this disastrous epidemic was, at times, coercive. In many instances, quarantines were instituted and people were banned from gathering in public places. Ordinances requiring the use of protective masks were widely and quickly passed. In some cases, such ordinances were briskly enforced.

But what is perhaps most startling about this worst of all modern mass casualty events is the relative paucity of public solicitude it engendered. People were far more concerned with the war in Europe, and so was the news media. Brutally afflicted Philadelphia, for instance, closed its schools, theaters, pool halls, and churches, but continued to conduct patriotic parades right through the worst of the epidemic.[6] On September 20, 1918, Camp Lewis, in the Puget Sound region of Washington state, reported 173 cases of influenza—yet this did not prevent 10,000 civilians from cramming together in the camp three days later to observe a review of the state's National Guard infantry.[7]

In San Francisco, there was much initial enthusiasm about the use of surgical masks. Ninety-nine percent of residents used them—even before the enactment of a mandatory mask ordinance.[8] Yet when the epidemic started to decline, so did mask use. Dr. William Hassler, chief of San Francisco's Board of Health, waged an aggressive media campaign emphasizing the continuing importance of masks; police power was appropriated, and hundreds were arrested—all to no avail. Dissenters invoked their civil liberties, and eventually the ordinance suffered what Crosby characterizes as the "worst of possible fates . . . it became funny." Clever violations of the mask law became as fashionable as sneaking alcohol would be in a future era of Prohibition. Even Hassler was caught without a mask.[9] When another wave of influenza broke out at year's end, efforts to engender mask use failed outright—this time 90 percent of San Franciscans ignored Mayor Rolph's call for voluntary masking.[10]

The 1918 influenza epidemic starkly illustrates several sociological barriers to effective public health practice in mass casualty events, including the tendencies of the general public (1) to fear violent or exotic dangers (such as aggression from Germany or biological attacks) over natural or familiar dangers (such as influenza epidemics and motor vehicle accidents),[11] (2) to quickly acclimatize to specific dangers with subsequent dissipation of fear or concern, and (3) to prefer liberty and convenience over protection from mundane threats to health. These factors, combined with the tendency of the news media to focus on emerging violent and otherwise sensational threats, beget a skewed perception of risk among citizens at large. Fear of terrorism is a prime example. America could suffer terrorist-related losses of September 11th magnitude every month, perpetually, and the death toll would still not approach our mortality from motor vehicle accidents. Meanwhile, the same citizens who testify endlessly on television about their feelings of vulnerability to terrorism will drive home from their interviews at 75 miles per hour, two car lengths behind the potential victim in front of them.

Though public health workers may also fear exotic dangers more than familiar ones, this tendency is blunted by their attention to mortality data and other scientific indices of risk. What is striking about the 1918 influenza epidemic is the interventionist tendency of some public health authorities. This tendency is manifested in inclinations (1) to support coercive public health measures (such as the San Francisco mask ordinance) even when the public is willingly cooperating without coercion, (2) to feel that "something must be done" whenever public health is deteriorating—even if clearly effective measures are not readily available,[12] and (3) to underestimate public resistance to measures that infringe liberty.

Recent attempts by ethicists, legal authorities, and public health scholars to delineate the ethical and political conditions for legitimate public health interventions are in part a response to this public health interventionism (or at least to the perception of it). They are also, no doubt, efforts toward a strategy to secure public trust by advertising ethical restraints that limit intrusions by agents of public health. In this chapter we examine the ethical, political, and operational legitimization of coercion in mass casualty medicine, beginning with a seminal article by ten leading scholars in public health ethics.

GOOD REASONS LEGITIMACY

A legitimate use of coercion is one that appropriately integrates ethical, political, and scientific norms, given the particular context. Broadly speaking, there are two dimensions of legitimacy in the use of coercion. The first dimension—good reasons legitimacy (GRL)—is satisfied by well-formulated arguments that show how a proposed intervention makes ethical, political, and scientific sense. Practically speaking, this amounts to giving good reasons for the intervention. The second dimension—public justification legitimacy (PJL)—results from a process in which proposed interventions and their rationale are properly discussed, articulated, marketed, explained, or otherwise brought to life before the general public. As such, PJL involves both the application of (presumably democratic) procedural norms and a public sense that the norms have been applied in an authoritative way. These notions are linked in the notion of "legitimation" employed by political philosophers such as Jürgen Habermas.[13]

It is natural to assume that good reasons legitimacy precedes public justification legitimacy. After all, it would be folly to attempt to publicly explain or justify something without an argument or an inventory of good reasons. Even raising the issue of a possible intervention presumably involves some sort of prior cogitation. Why this particular intervention? Why now?

In "mapping the terrain" of public health ethics, scholars sponsored by the Green-wall Foundation recently focused on conflicts between "general moral considerations that are generally taken to instantiate the goal of public health—producing benefits, preventing harms, and maximizing utility—and those that express other commitments."[14] Of course, a prime example of a general moral consideration that expresses "other commitments" is the norm of avoiding coercion, which expresses the commitment to liberty and autonomy. The Greenwall scholars propose five "justificatory conditions" for public health interventions that infringe prima facie ethical norms such as the norm of avoiding coercion.

The first condition is "effectiveness," which applies when evidence or informed common sense indicate that a proposed infringement will probably serve public health in the intended manner. The application of this condition is largely scientific in nature; it depends more on an accurate account of the facts than on an ethical argument.

Second is "proportionality." A public health intervention is proportional when "the probable public health benefits outweigh the infringed general moral considerations." This issue hinges primarily on ethical considerations and will be discussed in more detail below.

Third and fourth are "necessity" and "least infringement," which involve, respectively, the right kind and the right degree of infringement. The right kind of infringement is that which is necessary to achieve a particular public health goal. Even if a given trade-off between public health and another ethical norm is proportional, that trade-off is not ethically justifiable if there is another way to produce the same benefit without violating the norm in question (and without violating another equally important norm). The right degree of infringement is that in which competing ethical norms are violated only as much as needed. As the authors note, "least infringement" may be viewed as a corollary of "necessity."

Finally, there is the condition of "public justification." This condition manifests the responsibility to "explain and justify" the moral infringement brought about by a public health intervention. The Greenwall scholars' account of this justificatory condition focuses on transparency in "offering moral reasons" for policy makers' decisions. In essence, it is conceived as the transfiguration of good reasons legitimacy (covered in the first four justificatory conditions) into public justification legitimacy. In their initial formulation, the authors do not require input from the affected parties as an element of public justification, but later in the paper they expand the notion of public justification into a prescription for "public accountability," which does require such input.

The Greenwall scholars are careful to note that they do not intend with these guidelines to articulate a universal ethic for public health. To the contrary, their guidance is meant to pertain specifically in the United States and sociopolitically similar contexts.[15] Nor do they claim that there is a consensus favoring any particular approach to public health ethics, even within the United States. "The terrain of public health ethics," they explain, "includes a loose set of moral concepts and norms that are variously called values, principles, or rules—that are arguably relevant to public health." The recognition of such concepts and norms "does not entail a commitment to any particular theory or method."[16]

In reality, things are even more unsettled in public health ethics than these admissions concede. To wit, the loose amalgam of public health ethical norms—such as those articulated in the Greenwall scholars five justificatory conditions—is so loose that it pretty much falls apart as soon as anyone tries to carve it into a useful tool for making ethical decisions. In establishing the "necessity" of a certain type of ethical infringement, for instance, one needs to ascertain that a public health good cannot be obtained without the proposed infringement or the infringement of another ethical norm that is equally or more important. Such a determination requires one to compare and contrast various non-public-health-related ethical commitments. In deciding whether it is better to require mustard gas victims to disrobe publicly for group decontamination, or to take control of a nearby hotel where decontamination can be accomplished in private showers,[17] one may need to ask: Is privacy more or less important than hotel owners' property rights? The answer, of course, depends on one's vision of the good and the right.

Attempts to establish proper proportionality between public health benefits and "other commitments" run into the same problem. As we observed in the previous chapter, the meaning and value of good health are highly contended. How, then, do we compare health protection and promotion to other values that are also subjects of intense disagreement? A central theme in democratic countries such as the United States is the commitment to freedom of conscience, manifested, for instance, in the tolerance of ethical pluralism and in the separation between church and state. But ethical pluralism implies a diversity of moral visions that precludes agreement on matters such as the proper proportion between health objectives and other ethical values. And the separation between church and state requires that no particular moral vision (no particular religious worldview and no particular secular moral ecology) shall be established or ensconced as the canonical political morality. Without a content-rich canonical political morality, it is difficult or impossible to authoritatively mediate the proportion between particular public health benefits and competing values. Rather than expecting good theorists or wise policy makers to solve such ethical problems with brilliant ethical analysis, democratic and ethically pluralistic polities like the United States depend on procedural standards that embody an array of well-established political values (such as rights to life, liberty, and the pursuit of happiness). But these well-established values, despite being fundamental and deeply held collective ethical commitments, beget little unanimity as to their ultimate justification, specification, and moral significance.

PUBLIC JUSTIFICATION LEGITIMACY

That is where public justification comes in. Though imbedded in authoritative political values, public justification is primarily procedural in nature. Public justification legitimacy (PJL), far from being a phenomenon in which policy makers enumerate good reasons for their exercise of power, is (or ought to be) a condition in which the standards for what counts in particular contexts as good reasons are appropriately deliberated, debated, and negotiated between policy makers and the general public. Because the array of moral visions in any particular ethically pluralistic jurisdiction shifts with emigration, immigration, conversion, and gradual changes in citizens' moral sensibilities, it is inevitable that decisional standards will also be in flux. What counts ethically as "good reasons" for intrusive public health measures will change with these shifting values. In a democracy, good reasons will always depend on (rather than dictate) the moral visions and the behavior of the general public.

The upshot is that, politically speaking, public justification legitimacy *precedes* good reasons legitimacy. Before one can enumerate, interpret, and balance all the reasons for a particular policy or intervention, one must first legitimize an inventory of reasons and establish a sense of how they should be integrated. That task requires public consultation. Even politically fundamental good reasons—such as constitutional principles and the "natural rights" of citizens articulated in the United States—are based on a prior public reckoning. In the Declaration of Independence, Thomas Jefferson and his coauthors maintain that the existence of natural rights to life, liberty, and the pursuit of happiness is a self-evident truth; and so is the equality of all men (presumably women as well). They proclaim: "We hold these Truths to be self-evident." But if they are really self-evident, why did the forefathers feel the need to declare that they "hold them" to be such? Doesn't self-evidence speak for itself? Michael Zuckert explains:

The language, the logic, and the historic connections of the Declaration all point to the same conclusion: the truths announced in the Declaration are not self-evident, nor are they pronounced to be. They are rather to be held as if self-evident within the political community dedicated to making them effective. The truths must serve as the bedrock or first principles of all political reasoning in that regime. While they stand as the conclusion of a chain of philosophical or scientific reasoning, they must stand at the beginning of all chains of political reasoning.[18]

Despite brilliant insight, Zuckert's account is incomplete in this passage. America's first principles were not merely the result of a chain of philosophical or scientific reasoning, or even of a multiplicity of distinct chains. They were an articulation of deeply held, emergent public values—"deeply held" in the sense that they enjoyed passionate, widespread approval; "emergent" in the sense that, despite their political primacy at a given point in time, they are products of social evolution that are provisional and hence revisable when values change substantially. In politics, even fundamental principles are subject to the human will.

The question for PJL becomes: What are the procedures and mechanisms that policy makers and political authorities should employ in consulting the public? Much of the response to this question is contained in state and federal constitutions that prescribe the practice of representative democracy. Ideally, citizens elect trustworthy representatives who offer the most appealing political "platforms." These platforms are, in large part, detailed interpretations of political values and how they ought to be converted into public policy. They emerge (again, ideally) from the dialectic between politicians and voters—an exchange that involves public opinion polls, debates, speeches, town hall meetings, and the like. When a politician serves the platform poorly, or when the platform falls out of favor by not delivering the expected results, reelection is less likely (unless the politician is able to develop a new and better platform). Certainly, then, the election cycles in representative democracies involve an important form of public consultation.

Another key element of representative democracy that facilitates orderly public input is the balance of powers. In the United States, the president is elected nationally and thus tends to have a platform that represents the overall "sense" of the national majority. Legislators are beholden to more localized jurisdictions and hence have an opportunity to represent interests that might be quashed by national campaigns with their inevitable leveling effect. The judiciary safeguards adherence to political procedures that facilitate public input, and its severance from direct public accountability helps protect minority interests from majoritarian bias (though, alas, the lack of accountability exacerbates judges' tendencies to inflict their own peculiar values).

For more than two centuries, this system has proved its mettle. Nevertheless, several well-known pitfalls limit the degree to which the electoral process and the balance of powers can satisfy aspirations for public participation. The first problem is the scope of services rendered, which has grown exponentially since the Constitution was ratified in 1789. As government influence is extended into more of society's workings, the sheer volume of issues and problems that confront elected officials has vastly outgrown their capacities to deal with them directly and competently. In the executive branch, regulatory departments have sprung up, operating for the most part without direct oversight from elected officials. In the legislature, panels are employed to research problems and recommend solutions. Neither the regulators, nor the panelists, nor various commission members who serve either branch of government are directly beholden to public values. In mass casualty medicine, most of the federal guidelines come from agencies such as the Centers for Disease Control (CDC), the Federal Emergency Management Agency (FEMA), the Department of Homeland Security, the Department of Defense (DOD), and many others. These agencies and departments are not staffed by elected officials. Public input into the ethical values that shape their guidelines is not guaranteed or optimized by the electoral process or the balance of power. Such is also the case with certain sources of federal funding for mass casualty medicine, which include relatively autonomous entities such as the Health Resources and Services Administration (HRSA) and the Agency for Healthcare Research and Quality (AHRQ).

Second, attempts to cultivate public input are hampered by the size and moral diversity of populations served. Even officials elected to the U.S. House of Representatives must balance conflicting ethical claims from large numbers of diverging moral communities and from individuals not deeply imbedded in any particular moral community. Public opinion polls and even community forums are blunt instruments for eliciting broad input in such jurisdictions. This problem is worse for senators and much worse for executive officials.

Third, diverging moral communities employ diverging moral vocabularies, which makes it difficult for politicians and policy makers to interpret public input. Members of different ethnic groups often draw from markedly different natural languages in expressing remarkably diverse ethical views, and there are cultural variations that vastly complicate simple ethnic classifications. Political ideology sometimes spans ethnic, class, and cultural boundaries but begets its own terminological confusion — witness the contrast between how welfare-state liberals and personal-responsibility libertarians understand such terms as "choice," "freedom," "opportunity," and "obligation." Even public opinion surveys are difficult to interpret due to the plurality of possible meanings of the questions and available answers. Thoughtful citizens should be puzzled over pollsters' use of terms such as "somewhat agree" or the implications of choosing it over "somewhat disagree" (one of these implies the other). And what is the difference between "strongly agree" and "agree"? Does agreeing without strongly agreeing imply that you think the statement in question gets the matter exactly right, but you don't much care anyway? What if the statement gets the matter almost but not quite exactly right? Technically, one must disagree with such statements.

These are just a few of the problems that complicate endeavors to coordinate government policy with public values. Each presents a serious hurdle for the public justification of coercion in MCM. Scope of services, for instance, is a tremendous problem for elected officials tasked with overseeing the construction of ethically legitimate isolation and quarantine guidelines for a national epidemic. Cultural diversity complicates discussions about whether or not chemical warfare victims may be forced to disrobe publicly. And ideological incongruities tend to paralyze attempts to attain public agreement about "just" penalties for health care workers who refuse to cooperate with authorities in a mass casualty event.

Such difficulties are as old as democracy itself, yet recently they have become central foci for a relatively new wave in political philosophy: the study of deliberative democracy. As Joshua Cohen notes, deliberative democracies are associations of persons for whom "free deliberation among equals is the basis of legitimacy."[19] Theories of deliberative democracy, like most other contemporary theoretical responses to the problem of ineradicable ethical pluralism, are second-order political theories—that is, they are theories that suggest procedures for mediating refractory conflicts between proponents of mutually exclusive first-order ethical or political theories (first-order theories are theories that inscribe relatively complete, substance-rich ethical or political worldviews), while remaining mostly agnostic about the prominent first-order theories held by parties they anticipate having to mediate.[20]

The fundamental presumption of all accounts of deliberative democracy is in line with our conclusion about the ascendancy of PJL: In the face of political controversy, dissenting parties should be allowed to air out their multitudinous opinions, arguments, insights, and proposed solutions; and government agents should systematically take account of these offerings in their policy deliberations. Deliberative democrats also hold that citizens of deliberative democracies will (or should) regard decisions established through public deliberation as binding until they are revised through subsequent deliberation. In distinction to contractarians such as John Rawls and David Gauthier, deliberative democrats employ actual (rather than the ideal) deliberators. This policy imparts something of a "real world" air to many accounts of deliberative democracy—messy and uncomfortable, perhaps, for traditional political theorists, but provocative and promising for policy makers who need to make actual decisions about issues such as the use of coercion in mass casualty medicine.

Theories of deliberative democracy vary on factors such as (1) what counts as deliberation, (2) what counts as an acceptable result of political deliberation, (3) what methods of deliberation best facilitate acceptable results, and (4) why deliberation is preferable to other alternative mediating devices. In an attempt to sharpen our discussion of PJL, we will examine each of these factors.

DELIBERATIVE DEMOCRACY AND RATIONAL CONSENSUS

For the sake of manageable simplicity, theories of deliberative democracy can be lumped into two general categories. The first and most prominent category I will call "rational consensus theory" (RCT). For RCT, public deliberation is rational argumentation between participants who offer mutually acceptable reasons as premises. Substantial moral consensus (i.e., consensus about how things ought to be) is both a necessary condition and an anticipated product. The second category is what I will call "modus vivendi theory" (MVT), which describes public deliberation as open-ended, problem-centered dialogue. Though it too is based to some degree on moral consensus (i.e., consensus supporting the procedures it employs), the only further consensus it expects—and its only explicit objective—is consensus about a particular course of action. Often this result will take the form of a political compromise.

Rational consensus theory harks back to the Enlightenment, with its focus on reason and rationality. Because of this focus, RCT views deliberation in the Enlightenment way, as an exercise in rationality. RCT prescribes argumentation and expects that arguers will employ premises that are accessible to other arguers—accessible, that is, in the sense that everyone in the deliberating group can accept them as prima facie plausible on the basis of scientific evidence, rational insight, or collective belief.[21] For the most part it eschews other sources of conviction, such as religious insight, sectarian tradition, loyalty, or emotional response (these being too idiosyncratic to facilitate moral consensus, and perhaps too visceral to count as rational).

The mutually acceptable reasons constraint acts, in RCT, as a kind of wall between public and private domains. By excluding religious speech and sectarian principles, proponents of RCT hope to carve a relatively neutral public language or lingua franca that is based on science, reason, and whatever degree of "overlapping consensus" they can obtain. The concept of overlapping consensus and its variants is crucial, since science and reason alone don't go very far in the establishment of a public vocabulary. John Rawls, who combines contractarianism with tentative commitments to RCT, presents four crucial features of an overlapping consensus.

First, it involves overlapping content from reasonable (as opposed to "unreasonable or irrational") doctrines. This means that RCT views itself, not as a response to the concrete reality of ethical pluralism—which involves complex interplay between reason, tradition, superstition, bias, and other messy motives—but rather as a response to theoretical conundrums and partings of the way. Rawls writes: "The crucial fact is not the fact of pluralism as such, but of reasonable pluralism."[22]

Second, an overlapping consensus is freestanding and independent of the reasonable doctrines whose overlapping content comprise it. In this respect, it purports to preserve tolerance for reasonable ethical and metaphysical disagreements without arbitrarily inflicting a particular worldview.

Third, an overlapping consensus is a moral consensus, with a moral object and moral grounds. The object of the consensus—political conceptions, principles, ideals, and practices—is moral in the sense that it manifests views about what is right and good. The grounds are moral because they reside in particular reasonable ethical doctrines that generate the overlapping content.

Fourth, an overlapping consensus is stable in the way that moral commitments are stable. It is valued, not merely for instrumental purposes, but also as an end in itself, and hence it will not be susceptible to revision as soon as there is a shift in the balance of powers between persons with competing comprehensive ethical worldviews.

A robust conception of overlapping consensus of the sort prescribed by Rawls begets a hard-and-fast distinction between public and private morality. It creates this distinction by employing its inventory of shared reasonable values as a taxonomical device. Public morality is founded on shared reasonable values and speaks solely in the language of these values. Private morality is whatever countervails or falls outside the scope of these fundamental public values. To function effectively as a basis for public morality, the overlapping consensus must be robust enough to provide resources for a public vocabulary, yet limited enough to allow for legitimate moral diversity. One of the primary aims of deliberation, according to rational consensus theory, is to enhance and rationalize public life by augmenting the moral consensus.

A problem with all of this is that it deviates radically from what actually occurs, and what reasonably might be expected to occur, in public dialogue. When it comes to public debate, we can expect neither pure practical reason, nor purity of heart, nor orderliness of procession to carry the day. Several factors preclude such optimistic projections. First, if dialogue is to be free and uncoerced, as most delibera-tivists insist,[23] then citizens must be free *not* to participate. Those who care the most about a given issue, those with resources and confidence in their ability to make a difference, and those with the most firmly held opinions tend to self-select and may consequently comprise the bulk of participants. Such parties will tend to be more interested in being heard than in hearing others. They will cajole and denounce, shout and bear witness; and they will seek consummation of their deepest interests and commitments before they will submit to the ardor and frustration of reasoned discourse.

For the most part, public exhortations will be gilded with a veneer of self-righteousness. Iris Marion Young, for instance, has argued for activism over deliber-ation, explaining that "the activist believes it important to express outrage at contin-ued injustice, in order to motivate others to act." Nowhere does she betray even a tinge of self-doubt regarding her version of justice. Nor does she condone inclusive discussion about the meaning of concepts like justice. To the contrary, her activist "finds laughable the suggestion that he and his comrades should sit down with those whom he criticizes, and whose policies he opposes, to work out an agreement through reasoned argument they all can accept. The powerful officials have no motive to sit down with him, and even if they did agree to deliberate, they would have the power to steer the course of the discussion."[24]

Even if her version of activism is less potent than she thinks, Young makes an important criticism of RCT. As a matter of basic sociology and the psychology of per-suasion, the appeals in RCT to solidarity, other-spiritedness, and the rule of reason are not likely to prevail. James Madison was more realistic, I think, than most con-temporary deliberative democrats when he reflected that the causes of faction are "sown in the nature of man," and "everywhere brought into different degrees of ac-tivity, according to the different circumstances of civil society."[25] In like fashion, Young looks warily for rational consensus, and rarely finds it.

Madison (in the above-cited essay) makes another important point that chal-lenges the feasibility of deliberative democracy fashioned according to RCT. The forces creating faction and dissensus are powerful, and they are nurtured by liberty. Because of their virility, it is unlikely that democracies could achieve the kind of robust overlapping consensus required by RCT to establish its ethical lingua franca and its deliberative practices, and it is even more unlikely that free and open discus-sion would produce deeper levels of consensus. For Madison, it is sufficient to pro-cure enough agreement to implant a federal constitution.

Now recall that overlapping consensus, on Rawls' account, must be robust enough to beget a public morality, yet limited enough to allow for ethical pluralism and tolerance. Rawls refers to James Madison's version of public consensus as "constitutional consensus" and laments that it is too substance-poor to support his version of the just society.[26] But if Madison and contemporary thinkers of his ilk are right, Rawls will not and cannot ever achieve his more robust objective. In fact, even Rawls admits that there is no overlapping consensus about justice in the United States such as his doctrine of justice as fairness requires and that estimating the prospects for such a consensus is a speculative venture.[27]

It is beyond the scope of this book to debate at length the empirical probabilities for deliberation on the RCT model. Though I think they are prohibitively slight, my central focus is on the issue of whether or not RCT, even if achievable, presents a desirable option for contemporary democracy. I do not think that it does, and I will argue for the alternative, modus vivendi theory (MVT).

MODUS VIVENDI

A *modus vivendi* is a working arrangement between contending parties that allows them to live or work together peacefully in spite of intractable differences. As a political vision, modus vivendi is characterized by (1) its fundamental objective of obtaining political stability and peace, (2) its indifference to particular conceptions of the good and right, (3) its esteem for permission and consent, and (4) its strategies of balancing power and facilitating compromise. As a preface to the practical concept of public justification legitimacy that I employ for the remainder of this book, I will briefly elaborate each of these characteristics and suggest how they are an improvement over the tenets of rational consensus theories.

Most modus vivendi theorists trace their lineage back to Thomas Hobbes. In distinction to subsequent liberal theorists such as John Locke and John Stuart Mill (but roughly in accordance with successors such as David Hume and James Madison), Hobbes repudiated the idea of founding political philosophy on a full-fledged ethical doctrine.[28] Hobbes recognized the existence of public morality, but he viewed it as the expression of a distinctive political will,[29] not as a universal morality or even necessarily the morality of individual citizens. For Hobbes, particular moralities will inevitably diverge, such that some form of moral toleration is needed within the state. While Locke defended toleration, at least in part, because it manifests the Protestant version of ethics he took the state to embody,[30] and Mill defended it because he thought it was dictated by utilitarian ethics, Hobbes viewed toleration primarily as a means of securing peace.[31] Hobbes was struck by the barbarity and contentiousness that arise in natural human interactions, and he focused his political vision on preventing violence by keeping contending forces in check.[32]

One need not be as pessimistic as Hobbes to endorse a modus vivendi approach to politics. As one neo-Hobbesian, Patrick Neal, has argued, there is nothing in the Hobbesian vision that precludes the cultivation of moral rules and sentiments in pre-political society or among citizens of a polity.[33] For Hobbes, basic political morality supervenes on prudence and is about all one can expect; but this view is a function of Hobbesian psychology and is in no respect required for adherents to modus vivendi political theory. Nor must one be sympathetic to Hobbes's prescription for an all-powerful sovereign—unless one is convinced that such is the best means for people to secure their own safety and well-being (a rare perspective in the West).

What is required is the recognition that differences between individuals and moral communities tend to be serious, explosive, and potentially violent and that security cannot be established on a foundation of moral consensus. That is what the proponents of rational consensus seem not to grasp. In this regard, Neal observes, rational consensus theorists

> overestimate the sources of stability provided by their neutrality models of justice. I think this happens because each tends to underestimate the coercive role of the state in their respective accounts of liberal justice and its attendant stability. Stability is seen, on their model, as arising from consensus at the level of *beliefs of citizens*. . . . This argument hinges on the underlying notion that whereas the modus vivendi model generates only prudential motivations for adherence, the neutrality model generates "moral" motives, which are, it is postulated, impervious to the distribution of power. . . . With regard to Rawls, for example, what is actually argued is the existence of a descriptive link or match between elements of individual's [sic] conceptions of the good and elements of the public conception of justice. But what is not explained is why the existence of that analytical link provides the individual with a motivation (moral or otherwise, for that matter) to adhere to the public conception. . . . I suggest that [the rational consensus theorists' view] is quite a sanitized understanding of the degree to which pluralistic conflict threatens social and political stability. . . . The picture connoted by formulations such as "disputes about the nature of the good life" and "alternative conceptions of the good" is a relatively benign and pacific one. . . . With our attention focused upon the fact that they disagree about the concrete answer to the question of the good life, it is easy to overlook just how much social order is implicitly being assumed when we suppose that *that* question is the root of conflict and the threat to stability. This is not a picture of people fighting over wealth, or power, or race, or ethnicity, or selfishness, or greed, or vainglory, or—well, just about anything people actually fight over in the real world.[34]

Neal may overstate the case by implying that moral motives do not contribute significantly to political wrangling and instability. Debates over abortion, euthanasia, animal rights, and capital punishment belie that notion. His central point, however, is compelling. The moral motives that flow from a particular worldview are organically imbedded in a matrix of passions, prejudices, desires, and fears.[35] These forces merge tenaciously in the human will and cannot be tweaked apart and redirected by savvy political philosophers. For the most part, we must work with what we have, snatching ethical insight and progress where the situation allows. In the meantime, stability and safety are pressing concerns.

Rational consensus theorists who optimistically presume that erudition and careful deliberation will quickly and peacefully settle moral controversies are at odds with the fundamental datum their theories are designed to address—the reality and intractability of ethical pluralism. In this failure, they also turn a blind eye to the extent to which their own schemes hinge on the threat of force. It would be better to address the problem of coercion directly and be clear as to where it is or is not needed to ensure social stability and peace.

The focus on stability and peace in modus vivendi theory is a function not merely of the perception that moral and political controversies are complex and dangerous; MVT also holds that they are intractable. In *Justice Is Conflict,* Stuart Hampshire initiates his defense of MVT by stating that "justice cannot consist of any kind of harmony or consensus either in the soul or in the city, because there never will be such a harmony, either in the soul or in the city."[36] Bioethics' most visible proponent of modus vivendi, H. Tristram Engelhardt Jr., dedicates the first two chapters of his seminal treatise, *The Foundations of Bioethics,* to exposing the ineradicable nature of moral pluralism and the inevitable failure of all projects—past, present, and future—to overcome it with reason.[37]

Both of these thinkers suggest that the quest for peaceful mediation of moral controversies has requirements so indelible that they may be regarded as transcendental conditions for secular morality.[38] Engelhardt states this thesis explicitly in defending his principle of permission (examined below).[39] For Hampshire, the content of the requirement and its justification are much the same as Engelhardt's: "My requirement from my moral enemies is the requirement that I impose upon myself: that contrary views of what is just and fair are allowed equal hearing, equal access, in the city or state, and that no one conception of substantial justice in society is imposed by domination and by the threat of force."[40] He goes on to claim that the authority and justification for this requirement "are to be found in the structure of practical reason itself." This thesis, he observes, is based on "a kind of transcendental argument."[41]

What is clear for modus vivendi theory—whether or not we accept the transcendental qualifications—is that the intractability of moral pluralism demands that a polity remain indifferent to its prominent, competing, content-full conceptions of the good and right. The state cannot reasonably, fairly, or safely mediate moral controversy by arbitrarily inflicting a particular morality that is not shared by the public at large. Hence, the milquetoast state tolerance of most contemporary liberal polities—which supports a limited but compulsory form of diversity as a positive value internal to the state ethos—is largely replaced by what John Gray has termed "the radical tolerance of indifference."[42]

The radical tolerance of indifference, as a property of state institutions and procedures, is manifested in the refusal to use coercion to sanction a particular moral perspective at the expense of other prominent competing perspectives. As a property of citizens or of politicians, the "tolerance of indifference" is something of a misnomer, since individuals are not required to regard others' moral views indifferently. To the contrary, they are free to loath and publicly condemn their fellow citizens' behaviors and beliefs. But citizens are expected to be indifferent in one crucial respect: they must strictly respect others' politically established rights, even when these are exercised in ways they find heinous.

The indifferent state is not a neutral state. Gray and most other MVT proponents acknowledge the state's prerogative to sanction some degree of "formative project" (i.e., cultivation of civic habits vital to political life), but this prerogative is sharply limited and mostly confined to the endorsement of a thin repertoire of virtues that actually elicit consensus approval. For the most part, the state will tolerate even the most despicable opinions, biases, and prejudices. Coercive state intervention is necessary only in particular cases where such reprehensible orientations lead to violence or to other abridgements of political rights. Civic morality in the indifferent state might be robust; but it will not be robust because it is coerced.

In maintaining its indifference, the state is not endorsing ethical relativism (the view that there are no objectively defensible standards of the good and right). Nor is the modus vivendi state based on value pluralism (the view that there are many incompatible conceptions of the good that are objectively defensible and ethically legitimate).[43] Some modus vivendi theorists (Hampshire and Gray, for instance) are value pluralists; some are not (Engelhardt and the present author, for instance). What they have in common is that they believe that general rational consensus in favor of a single comprehensive vision of the good and/or the right (or even consensus on a rough approximation of such) is neither a plausible nor a legitimate objective of the state, at least in the foreseeable future. For this reason, MVT prescribes the radical tolerance of indifference.

To be radically tolerant tautologically implies restraint in nondefensive uses of force. Consequently, all modus vivendi theorists insist on some sort of principle of consent or permission; and all of them insist that this principle is the sole or primary basis for legitimate state coercion. When someone attacks us without our (direct or indirect) consent, we and the state are justified in resisting—by force if necessary. However, when we consent to a certain political project, institution, or rule, the state has the prerogative to coerce our compliance.

We've already viewed Hampshire's principle of consent in the passage above. Undeniably, it is vague as to the precise requirements for public input into state actions that might involve coercion, and his subsequent writing does not sharpen the picture appreciably. Clearly, he believes that every moral community should be heard—by mechanisms that will vary between jurisdictions. He also holds that substantive moral visions should not be coercively foisted on citizens. What remains to be worked out—Hampshire leaves this task to others because he does not think it admits of a universal recipe—is just who precisely must give consent, in which circumstances, by which procedures.

Engelhardt is more explicit on these matters. His principle of permission is formally expressed in the following terms:

> Authority for actions involving others in a secular pluralist society is derived from their permission. As a consequence:
>
> i. Without such permission or consent there is no authority;
>
> ii. Actions against such authority are blameworthy in the sense of placing the violator outside the moral community in general, and making licit (but not obligatory) retaliatory, defensive, or punitive force.
>
> A. Implicit consent: individuals, groups, and states have authority to protect the innocent from unconsented-to force.
>
> B. Explicit consent: individuals, groups, and states can decide to enforce contracts or create welfare rights. . . .
>
> E. Public policy implications: the principle of permission provides moral grounding for public policies aimed at defending the innocent. . . .
>
> G. The principle of permission grounds what can be termed the morality of autonomy as mutual respect.[44]

Persons, in Engelhardt's political sense, are defined by their ability to give or deny consent.[45] Engelhardt endorses a basically Lockean theory of the acquisition of property and income, and holds that taxes can be collected in accordance with the Lockean proviso.[46] With the consent of those who will pay, taxes for welfare benefits and other entitlements is also consistent with the principle of permission. Taxes without consent are a violation of the principle of permission and justify resistance when states exercise force to collect them.

For the purposes of this study, we will accept Engelhardt's formal account of the principle of permission. However, one clarification and one revision of Engelhardt's interpretation are necessary. The clarification regards loci of permission. In the above formulation, Engelhardt lists "individuals, groups and states" as permission-giving entities. Since there are possible antagonisms between these sources, guidance is needed to align particular sources of permission with their proper contexts. Though it is tempting to designate individual persons as the sole legitimate sources of permission across all contexts, in practice this norm is hardly realistic. Broad measures such as the construction of highways and disaster plans or the ratification of constitutions would be impossible if every individual retained veto rights. The most straightforward alternative is to acquire individuals' permission to transfer a limited inventory of permission-giving and veto rights to particular moral communities or political entities. This idea operated in 1787, at the Federal Convention in Philadelphia, where representatives from the various states met to construct a federal constitution that would replace the Articles of Confederation. Here even the state representatives were inclined to relinquish particular permission-giving rights. Every state but Maryland agreed that ratification by a minimum of nine states would bind all the rest.[47]

A revision of Engelhardt's interpretation of the principle of permission is necessary because his theory of property is too facile. The concept of property is a social construct with a basis in and implications for morality, well-being, and the justification for coercion. As such, it too must be regarded as a modus vivendi, susceptible to the principle of permission. Contemporary legal and philosophical doctrines of the acquisition of property are complex, but to apply the modus vivendi approach they should be regarded as a starting point. The upshot is that the application of MVT in the context of the United States will have an attenuated libertarian flavor — but not as libertarian as the theory elaborated by Engelhardt, and not necessarily libertarian in the economic sense.[48] On the broad view, the modus vivendi approach can beget a variety of political and economic structures. Hampshire, for instance, favors socialism.[49]

Proponents of rational consensus theory will criticize the American version of MVT for perpetuating injustice. In one sense, this criticism is accurate, even with respect to the specific libertarian brand of procedural justice that MVT would approve in the United States. To wit, the prominent, quasi-Lockean conception of just property acquisition that holds sway in this country has not been satisfied by many property owners.[50] In a deeper sense, however, this objection is untenable. Substantive principles of justice are just the kind of thing that are at stake in the modus vivendi republic, and just the sort of thing that RCT fails most miserably in establishing. Rational consensus liberals have no basis for imposing such principles when they cannot show that they are objects of rational consensus.

In the current social and political milieu, the only legitimate principle of social justice is a procedural principle based on the principle of permission. If power and property is shown to be illegitimate on the tenets of this principle, corrections should be made. Beyond such remedies, however, there is no recourse for contemporary deliberators but to begin where we are. MVT becomes a question of strategy.

COMPROMISE

Recall two strategies offered by modus vivendi theory: balancing powers and facilitating compromise. For the former, much credit is due James Madison, who developed Montesquieu's doctrine of countervailing powers and helped express it in the U.S. Constitution near the end of the eighteenth century. The manifestation of this doctrine in three branches of the federal government has already been described and hardly needs further elaboration. In the next chapter, balancing powers will be relevant in our discussion of agency. For now, however, we will focus on the strategy with the most direct bearings on the conduct of deliberation: facilitating compromise.

Rational consensus theorists, as we observed, hunger for ordered discourse between mutually congenial parties, aimed at forging a canon of authoritative values that will render large swaths of humanity into a single cohesive political community. Modus vivendi theorists, on the other hand, are lax on rules of discourse, guarded about congeniality, and absolutely bereft of hope or aspirations for a morally robust political canon. If the modus vivendi thinker tingles over thoughts of a global community or universal peace, she nevertheless will restrain herself from believing that such ideals can be accomplished through rational consensus about the right or the good. She knows that compromise, not consensus, is the grease that lubricates political machinery.

Virtually every modus vivendi theorist has argued on behalf of compromise.[51] Within their ranks, there is a distinct consensus about it. A political compromise is a provisional agreement, by mutual concession, about what *will* be done, undertaken by parties who disagree about what *ought* to be done or about what they'd optimally *prefer* to do. What *will* be done is, from the perspective of each party, the best mutually workable approximation of their top choice, given the fact that they have been unable to bring other parties around to their view.

Suppose there is a disaster preparedness meeting in O'Fallon, Illinois, between the mayor, the fire chief, and the CEO of the nearest hospital (of course, other parties would need to be invited, but we will keep the example simple). The agenda includes decisions about the distribution of antibiotics in a serious epidemic, public provision of a newly FDA-approved vaccine for anthrax,[52] and the delivery of nonemergency medical care in public health emergencies. After assessing relevant data, various guidelines, and so forth, and discussing ethical, legal, logistical, and political issues, three points of contention arise. First, regarding the distribution of antibiotics for potentially exposed patients: the mayor favors a first-come, first-served protocol; the fire chief favors a protocol that prioritizes public employees and their families; and the CEO wants to prioritize essential personnel such as EMTs, nurses, and physicians but make no special allowance for their families. Second, regarding the vaccine: the mayor wants to offer unlimited voluntary immunization immediately; the fire chief favors mandatory immunization of all citizens; and the CEO thinks that vaccines should be withheld. Third, regarding nonemergency medical care in public health emergencies: the mayor favors the expansion of surge capacity in hospital facilities and medical clinics so that they can serve as sites for such care; the fire chief recommends secondary assessment centers (SACs); the CEO recommends modest increases in surge capacity, compatible with available public funding, coupled with the utilization of mobile medical clinics. Some of these differences reflect diverging ethical beliefs (for instance, the mayor's antibiotic distribution scheme reflects his strict egalitarian tendencies, and the CEO's scheme reflects her utilitarian beliefs). Many of the positions (e.g., the fire chief's antibiotic distribution scheme and the CEO's opinion on expanding surge capacity) reflect particular loyalties and professional commitments. And sometimes the differences are based on diverging opinions on the degree of threat (e.g., the opinions on immunization) or what will work (e.g., the fire chief's favoritism for SACs versus the CEO's preference for mobile medical clinics).

Each party is committed to deciding on a policy package that everyone is willing to approve, but it is evident that this objective cannot be reached merely on the basis of persuasive argument. Several compromise packages are suggested and debated, and the prospect of no action (i.e., sticking with the current provisions—ad hoc distribution of antibiotics, immunization voluntarily through doctor's appointments, and routine medical care through the usual channels) is also discussed. In the end, the group decides that (1) antibiotics will be distributed according to the mayor's first-come, first-served scheme; (2) no action will be taken on the vaccines; and (3) surge capacity will be enhanced only to the degree possible given available funds, with overflow routine medical care provided at secondary assessment centers for non-transmissible illnesses and by mobile medical clinics for transmissible illnesses.

Each party has made concessions, and each still believes that there are better options than the adopted package. But each also believes that this is close as they can possibly get (given the others' contrary views) to an optimum package, and furthermore, that the adopted package is better than no action at all. The mayor sacrifices serious political capital in committing the city to SACs and to the provision of mobile clinics, but he is very happy with the policies on antibiotic distribution and immunizations. The fire chief knows that the antibiotic scheme will cause anxiety for firefighters. However, he takes solace in the fact that he can probably successfully urge personnel under his command to get the vaccine (and they will be happy about having a choice). He, like the CEO, is relatively sanguine about the plan for routine medical care, though both think it will be something of a logistical nightmare. The CEO is satisfied about protecting her hospital from massive expenses in the provision of immunizations and routine medical care, but remains uneasy about the likely deleterious side effects that will attend large-scale use of the vaccine for a threat she considers remote. She also is worried about the loss of crucial personnel who do not get antibiotics on an expeditious basis. The parties have consented to a compromise, and despite the mixed feelings, they leave knowing they have done their best to serve their organizations and community.

The political compromise in this example establishes a modus vivendi. Neat formulations of substantial justice and other ethical principles are not in evidence. Moral consensus is sparse and elusive (though not entirely absent). And progress is made.

Two other features of compromise-ready MVT also commend it over RCT: it avoids polarization into two parties, and it impedes the tendency toward an oligarchy of experts and other elites. By the former, I mean that compromise-ready deliberation is something of a preventative against the coalescence of consensus-oriented discussants into two mutually contending parties. By the latter, I refer to the tendency of compromise-oriented deliberation to forestall oligarchic weak consensus (a consensus of powerful elites that is coercively imposed on a target population that does not share in the consensus).[53]

When moral consensus is the aim, discussants are presented with the impossible task of reaching agreement about issues that generate substantial controversy. Compromise becomes necessary, but it must be done covertly in order not to shatter the illusion of consensus. What happens is that antagonistic discussants consolidate (through internal compromise) into ostensibly unified groups. Differences within the group are then publicly minimized for the sake of a unified front. Instead, everyone focuses on "common ground." This process of consolidation continues, as each party attempts to recruit as many partners as possible in efforts to thwart what they view as the most threatening countercoalition. Eventually, the dynamics of power dictate that there will be only two major contending parties, each campaigning to achieve a majority great enough to legitimately proclaim that they represent the consensus beliefs of the combined group (or, as in national politics, of the population at large). Paradoxically, then, efforts at moral consensus breed adversarial politics.

Simple majoritarian democracy is a classic case, in that it inevitably begets efforts to proclaim a consensus ethos and always quickly devolves into adversarial duality or cultural tyranny. Writing in the early nineteenth century, John Calhoun accurately predicted that the trend to majoritarian democracy would produce polarization in U.S. politics and the entrenchment of a two-party system based precisely on these kinds of considerations. His alternative—"concurrent democracy"—is a modus vivendi vision. Concurrent democracy "regards interests as well as numbers—considering the community as made up of different and conflicting interests, as far as the action of the government is concerned; and takes the sense of each, through its majority or appropriate organ, and the united sense of all, as the sense of the entire community."[54] Calhoun contrasted compromise, the primary mechanism of his concurrent majority, with force, the inevitable tool of majoritarian democracy.[55] As the quoted passage indicates, Calhoun believed that concurrent democracy, despite (or rather because of) its recognition of diverging interests and beliefs, would create more harmony and unity than a simple majoritarian democracy. Concurrent democracy allows conflicting parties freely to debate and negotiate their differences, thus diluting the disappointment of compromise with the satisfaction of genuinely free collaboration. Majoritarian democracy (and all other efforts to quickly establish a content-rich morality by political means) also involves some degree of compromise; but in this case, the compromise is falsely advertised as consensus, then imposed through the threat of force. Because there is little free collaboration, there is little unity or solidarity.

Rational consensus theorists distinguish themselves from majoritarian democrats by their portrayal of deliberation—and its product, rational consensus—as a dignifying, harmonizing, edifying device. Deliberation to rational consensus is, for them, just the kind of "appropriate organ" that Calhoun would need to make concurrent majority work. It remedies adversarial duality or cultural tyranny, on their account, by (1) including everyone in the deliberations, (2) equalizing the power differential between discussants, and (3) distilling out deliberative content that is not "reasonable." But there are immense and insurmountable problems with each of these strategies.

The first strategy (inclusiveness) is commendable, insofar as it can be achieved without coercing people into participation, but it will do little or nothing to forestall polarization. The second strategy (power equalization) is largely a charade. Deliberative groups will always be stratified with respect to various sources of power and authority. Unsurprisingly, proponents of RCT construct a model that shifts power in their direction—that is, toward those who are trained in disputation and philosophical reasoning. Indeed, some power differentials seem worthy of universal condemnation (e.g., those resulting when employers are placed in small deliberative groups with employees), and many of these can be effectively controlled. But ambitious power-leveling schemes tend to base themselves on strategies (e.g., income redistribution) that beg the question on just the sort of matters that deliberation should be aimed at addressing.

The third strategy (distilling out content that is not "reasonable") involves the enforcement of rigorous rules of appropriate discourse or the creation of a neutral lingua franca. That strategy assumes, once again, that we know enough in advance about the right and the good to construct such an edifice of rules and vocabulary.[56] Such an assumption is nonsense. It is dangerous to democracy insofar as it uses the church/state division to exclude competing moral visions and establish the church of liberal humanism, or egalitarian cosmopolitanism, or whatever ethos its architects choose to incorporate into their deliberative structures. Furthermore, this approach virtually presumes the priority of good reasons legitimacy over public justification legitimacy by claiming extensive advance knowledge of what sort of thing should count as a good reason. We have already exposed the problems with such claims.

RCT frequently defends its emphasis on reason and convergence by employing a hard-and-fast distinction between deliberation proper and negotiation (the latter being prevalent in compromise).[57] Negotiation (or "bargaining," as the pejorative often goes) is regarded as distasteful because it involves fixed preferences and thus interferes with two crucial outcomes that make deliberative democracy attractive: the accumulation of ethical knowledge, and the enhancement of solidarity. But RCT, by imbedding its values in discourse structures, is guilty of just the kind of value fixation it purports to avoid. MVT, on the other hand, contains nothing that implies preferences will be fixed. To the contrary, peoples' preferences, moral inclinations, and loyalties will in many cases be more malleable when they are not countered by force. When given relatively free reign—as modus vivendi theory prescribes—these characteristics beget the psychic energy that good deliberation requires. Meanwhile, the implication from RCT theorists—that open-minded persons will insist on consensus and refuse to compromise—borders on the absurd.

RCT generally conceives the articulation of "common ground" as the starting point of deliberation, thinking that this positive focus will facilitate timely convergence. More often, it serves to divert attention from the fundamental problems that deliberation needs to address. In most instances (e.g., the O'Fallon example above), common ground is obvious. Though sometimes common ground can be fruitfully expanded—as, for instance, in surveying empirical data and clearing up divisive confusions—the navigation of moral controversy proceeds more quickly when the problem is clearly delineated.[58] The problem, in most cases, consists largely of incompatible ethical claims and/or clashing interests. Hence, Kevin Wildes, a bioethicist who propounds a form of modus vivendi theory, recommends that each moral community, in engaging moral controversies with other moral communities, should "seek to understand what binds it to others by first understanding how it differs from others."[59]

MODUS VIVENDI IN MASS CASUALTY MEDICINE

With respect to mass casualty medicine, the modus vivendi approach and its method of compromise are most useful at the public policy level, where deliberation is the source of public justification legitimacy (PJL). In an actual mass casualty event, on the other hand, there will often be precious little time for deliberation. Instead, good judgment must be exercised by the major actors. Good judgment is based on good reasons, which is to say, it expresses good reasons legitimacy (GRL).

As we observed, GRL about ethical matters in the pluralistic polis is dependent on prior deliberation. It is a function of PJL. When public officials, health care providers, and rescuers make urgent ethical decisions during disasters, they should, as far as possible, manifest values that have been approved in public deliberation. There is only one way to achieve such an objective: by incorporating publicly sanctioned values into MCM protocols and training. If the public values are not habituated through study and repetition, we cannot expect them to emerge on the front lines.

The Delaware tularemia scenario described in chapter 1 illustrates one way in which a disjunction between public and professional values occurs and is manifested. It represents a failure of coordination between public deliberation (i.e., by the Delaware legislature, presumably in concert with prior deliberation between representatives and constituents) and medical practice. Because Dr. Welby failed to internalize values the legislators thought they had inscribed, her actions were politically illegitimate. Part of the problem might have been with the inscription, and part of the problem might have resided in Dr. Welby herself. More often, such failures result from the inability to effectively bridge the gap between policy and training. They are failures of communication, coordination, and diligent preparation.

In the 1918 influenza epidemic, noncooperation with the San Francisco masking ordinances stemmed mostly from failures at the level of deliberation. Office holders and public health authorities took it upon themselves to fashion public policies without public input. They were slow to consult but quick to coerce. And their activist tendencies led them to intervene in ways that lacked a sound scientific basis.

The remedy might not be as difficult as it seems. We have enumerated a bewildering host of barriers to effective deliberation. Even the more action-ready modus vivendi approach may seem strenuous beyond practicality. But in mass casualty medicine there is a saving grace (nasty though its origins may be). The calamitous events that provide its context have a serious depolarizing effect. When conditions get very bad and thousands of lives are at stake, people tend to rally around the imperative to rescue and help their fellow humans. Effective, workable compromise, and even moral consensus, becomes far more feasible.

In order to flesh out our conception of public justification legitimacy, clarify its determinations in good reasons legitimacy, and show how it pertains in the justification of coercion in mass casualty medicine, we need to turn to specific questions about participation in deliberation—including its loci, epistemic warrants, and particular contexts—and about the systematic application of justificatory criteria in MCM preparedness and response. These issues hinge on identifying the roles, competencies, and values that should pertain to various agents involved in MCM; and in specifying these roles, competencies, and values in a way that effectively cultivates that crucial ingredient for success in MCM: adaptability. Our discussion of legitimacy has been long and abstract. For nonphilosophers, I suspect it has also been tedious. Happily, what follows is more concrete and more tangibly relevant to the practice of mass casualty medicine.

CHAPTER FOUR

Public Policy and the Role of Experts

Feelings of self-importance blossom in many settings, but disaster seems to beget an exceptional profusion. Consider the Muncie, Indiana, smallpox epidemic of 1893, in which twenty citizens died, a public health official was shot, and vainglorious experts caused more harm than good. Almost from the beginning, in August of that year, there was dispute over both the source of the epidemic and how best to manage it. Several out-of-towners, dissenting physicians, and "highly experienced" observers confidently proclaimed that the offending illness was not smallpox at all, but rather, the more benign "waterpox." This mistaken claim was trumpeted by the media. Some people believed it and died as a result. Some failed to take necessary precautions. And some stubbornly resisted coercive isolation—a conflict that led inevitably, as it must, to violence. Most of the local physicians got the diagnosis right. Yet their egos prevented them from contributing as much as they could.

At the height of the epidemic, local physicians met with a few politicians and favored community members to produce a set of rules that they expected public officials to enforce. Most of the rules were sensible, if debatable. Others were unrealistic—as, for instance, Rule 14: "We recommend that no person except nurse and physician be permitted to visit any sick person until it is certainly ascertained that they are not suffering from small-pox."[1] When some of their recommendations were not enforced, the physicians reconvened to issue a joint resolution absolving themselves of all responsibility for the impending catastrophe. Subsequent to this washing-of-hands, the epidemic quickly petered out.

As with San Francisco's response to the influenza epidemic of 1918, officials and experts in Muncie appealed to their own moral and practical intuition as justification for using force. From the standpoint of modus vivendi theory, this approach is problematic, since the legitimization of coercive public health interventions such as isolation and quarantine requires public consultation and some form of advance public affirmation. Specifying the precise mechanism for this public affirmation becomes the central problem for modus vivendi theory and practice.

Individual citizens are the most obvious and recognizable bearers of the right to give permission. But if individuals are the proper locus for permission, then coercion is fully legitimate only when each individual has voluntarily accepted, in advance, that under certain circumstances he or she should be coerced. There are unfortunately two very obvious and very important practical barriers to identifying individual persons as the sole legitimate permission givers, each discussed briefly in the preceding chapter. First, universal individual advance veto rights would preclude many sensible and widely popular cooperative ventures (such as building highways and ratifying constitutions). Second, the objective of getting everybody's input often proves to be unworkable—especially in exigent circumstances such as mass casualty events in which there is not time for it.

The first problem, then, for those who would enact government by modus vivendi, is the question of agency. Which are the appropriate individual, community, and organizational roles in deliberation, decision ratification, leadership, and enforcement? In this chapter, we examine the roles of experts and news media in public deliberation about coercion in mass casualty medicine. Then, in subsequent chapters, we will examine related agency issues including: (1) stakeholders' role in public deliberation, (2) leadership authority in strategic and tactical decisions about coercion, and (3) the authority to make and enact decisions for particular coercive actions.

EXPERTS' ROLE IN PUBLIC DELIBERATION

The Muncie epidemic wasn't unique in precipitating a coalescence of genuine and fanciful experts. Illness, disaster, violence, and other sudden, unexpected, and fearful disruptions elicit cries for help. There will always be well-wishers, opportunists, sages, and savants—clothed in erudition and poised to heed the summons. This dynamic is as natural as the impulse to understand. And it is a crucial matter for deliberation.

The first requirement of good deliberation seems to be that it is based on an accurate assessment of the facts. Relevant factual input includes medical/scientific information, demographic information, political/legal information, and sometimes integrative judgments about probabilities (as in surveying the most likely results of an intervention). Good clinical medicine, for instance, is increasingly judged by the degree to which it is evidence-based. As Mills and Spencer have observed, this imperative is not merely a dictum of competence, but it is believed by many to be the clinician's primary ethical imperative.[2] Evidence-based medicine (EBM) has become, in the eyes of some, an ethics of medicine.[3]

Esteem for evidence is not reserved for ordinary clinical medicine alone. There have also been calls for evidence-based disaster medicine,[4] and with them also calls for the agents of evidence—experts. Expertise, in disaster medicine as elsewhere, is the preferred medium of evidence-based decision making. Scientific experts are those who are publicly recognized as possessing the training, knowledge, and skill required to frame, interpret, and apply evidence. Contemporary mass casualty medicine—even more than its counterpart of one hundred or so years ago when smallpox, yellow fever, and cholera threatened large swaths of humanity—is an affair for experts. Just as EBM has become a morality for many medical experts, so too is evidence-based disaster medicine a potential source of ethical norms for experts in disaster medicine.

Like ordinary EBM, evidence-based disaster medicine comes with an inventory of fundamental values. Mills and Spencer delineate three that pertain in ordinary contexts: (1) appropriate use of the best available research evidence, (2) appropriate appeals to experience, and (3) integration of individual patient values and preferences into clinical decisions. To this list we need to add a fourth value—important in all EBM, but especially in evidence-based MCM—integration of community values and preferences.

As Mills and Spencer argue, the values underlying EBM do not cohere seamlessly. One source of advocacy for the first value is the (economic and practical) need for clinical efficiency. Efficiency feeds on standardization, and the best standards are presumably tied to the best evidence. Unfortunately, both clinical experience and patient values can oppose standardization. What is best for a statistically generic member of a population may not be best for a particular patient.[5] Likewise, in disaster medicine, what is best for typical communities or jurisdictions may not be best for any specific community.

This dilemma presents a *strategic question* for evidence-based mass casualty medicine: How can we construct a disaster system that integrates best evidence with other crucial values? The danger of straightforward evidence-based MCM is that it will devolve into a mechanical, recipe-laden routine that ignores clinical experience, particular patient needs, and most importantly, fundamental social and political values that are specific to afflicted communities. There is also a related *tactical question*: When do clinical judgment, patient values, and/or community values trump evidence-based guidelines? This section addresses the strategic question on two levels: as a problem for experts who fashion MCM guidelines, and as a problem for policy makers who incorporate MCM guidelines into actual disaster systems. Our task amounts to an evaluation of the proper role of experts in deliberation about MCM.

The appeal to best research evidence is an appeal to facts—shorn as much as possible from the baggage of particular contingent human values. As we earlier observed, facts and values are not entirely discrete. They are mixed together in various combinations like two sides of a coin, except that in the case of facts and values one side might be a lot more robust than the other. We say, for instance, that factually speaking, the best way to catch a large brown trout in late afternoon at Lake Taneycomo is to dead drift a #18 midge pupa about a foot from the bottom. But this fact is to some degree a function of an angler's values. Some anglers prefer cast-and-lifting with Wooly Buggers, and they practice this technique so thoroughly that they can take more trout this way than with dead-drifted pupae. And some anglers, for similar reasons, will be more successful with spinning gear. Perhaps future anglers will choose to pursue scuba diving techniques—and harvest even greater quantities of brown trout.

Likewise in medicine, our choices of what techniques to practice and investigate, which outcomes to optimize, and which clinical trade-offs make the most sense are value manifestations that indelibly structure every form of clinical evidence. Even standards of statistical significance contain arbitrary value elements. Somewhere, sometime, somebody decided that less than a 5 percent probability that observed variations are caused by random chance is sufficiently small to declare that the variations are statistically (and hence, scientifically) significant. Upon this arbitrary estimate of the proper equilibrium between the desire for certitude and the need for scientific progress, a great divide has been constructed: on one side we have laudable, objective scientific facts; on the other, mere speculations. But despite the appeal of evidence and objectivity, there *are* no pristine facts—which is to say, we can never progress to the extreme fact-ward pole of the spectrum between facts and values.

Still, the pursuit of objectivity and factuality is possible and useful. Some claims really are primarily factual in nature ("rust is iron oxide"), just as some claims are primarily valuations ("courage is laudable"). Likewise, some statements are more objective than others. Objectivity involves amenability to observation, verification, and interpretation by other inquirers. It manifests in canons of study design, significance testing, and evidence-based medical practice—important devices, even given that these standards are limited in the degree of objectivity they can render.

Most useful clinical and MCM guidelines contain large dollops of both fact and value. It is important to recognize this generality, for scientific experts often confuse and exploit their audiences when they present fact-value amalgams as simple facts. In his contrarian study of disaster planning, Lee Clarke examines several such cases. One theme in Clarke's work is that tenuously supported fact claims that cohere with experts' values or worldviews often get bandied about until they become accepted as established or "scientific" facts. Clarke describes a multibillion dollar 1980s attempt by federal authorities—particularly the Federal Emergency Management Agency (FEMA)—to construct a crisis relocation plan for Americans undergoing an all-out nuclear attack. In their efforts to convince a skeptical public that such planning is worth the time and money, federal officials repeatedly stated that, with proper planning and good (but not flawless) execution, 80 percent of the population of the United States could survive a maximum-intensity nuclear war.[6] Where, Clarke asks, did such an idea come from? Apparently it was output from limited computer simulations based on a number of questionable and sometimes downright unreasonable assumptions.[7] The tenuous 80 percent number was quoted so frequently—not only by federal agents but eventually also by congresspersons, news media, and outside "experts"—that it eventually was accepted as an established fact. Thus, a high-level official opined: "Computer analyses have confirmed the *obvious.* Expected survival in large-scale nuclear attacks approximates 80 percent of the U.S. population, assuming good, but not perfect, evacuation in all U.S. risk areas prior to attack."[8]

Sometimes scientific experts presume that their (often exaggerated) knowledge of how to compute probabilities endows them with the ability to establish thresholds for value-laden concepts such as "acceptable risk." In this regard, Clarke describes an attempt by Long Island Lighting Company (LILCO) to justify the construction of a nuclear power facility on Long Island. This effort was eventually confounded by LILCO's inability to convince state and local officials, as well as citizens of Long Island, that they could quickly evacuate the at-risk population in the event of a nuclear accident. LILCO constructed an evacuation plan and attempted to demonstrate its practicability by conducting exercises. But several obstacles prevented them from pulling this off. First, LILCO was unable to enlist the participation of key state, county, and local officials (including the police), who considered the plan to be so implausible as to not warrant their time; and LILCO didn't even try to include such key participants as the news media and ordinary citizens. Second, many of the participants performed so poorly that confidence was undermined. Third, the exercises were premised on assumptions (e.g., that bus drivers would uniformly report for duty) that were based on tenuous analogies to more well-studied disaster phenomena (e.g., health care providers and professional responders typically reporting for duty).[9]

LILCO enlisted a cadre of experts, including federal agents, to argue that these exercises, interpreted in light of scientific knowledge about disaster response, demonstrated the adequacy of the evacuation plan. To the contrary, however, the exercises raised more problems than they solved. There was little scientific evidence that clearly pertained to their specific plan, and what evidence there was did not go very far in supporting it. In the end, proponents of the nuclear facility relied on two major strategies: (1) inventing a "realism doctrine" that held that, in an actual emergency, dissenting local authorities and citizens, who now considered the evacuation plan to be foolhardy, would nevertheless act in accordance with it, since they would be forced to regard it as the best and most reasonable option; and (2) claiming that apparent affinities between nuclear meltdown and less fearful disasters (e.g., floods) provided significant evidence that their proposal entailed acceptable risks, then shifting the burden of proof to opponents. Clarke writes: "LILCO's claim that its opponents' position was not supported by evidence was a claim of a different kind. It said that the opponents were depending more on ideology (where pure belief is paramount) than on science (where evidence is paramount) to support their case. This was a tricky argument to make given that LILCO also had no evidence for its position."[10]

With both the 80 percent survivability thesis (from the nuclear war scenario) and LILCO's claim that its evacuation scheme adequately controlled nuclear risks, political agendas and wishful thinking are disguised as scientific facts. In each scenario there is an assumption that estimates of acceptable risk are scientific problems best handled by experts. But such is not the case. Sometimes, as Clarke argues, actual risks are ineradicably obscure—they are not risks but uncertainties. In such cases, the conversion from uncertainty to risk is basically a rhetorical one, not an affair for objective science. However, even when risks can be determined with relative accuracy, the notion of acceptable risk remains unresolved. Acceptable risk hinges on human values, not neutral facts. Risks that are acceptable for one individual, or one moral community, may not be acceptable for the next.

Despite its immense potential value, scientific expertise does not beget expertise about values. For this reason there is an increasing tendency to consult ethicists on value issues related to public policy. Indeed, bioethicists and other practical ethicists may have extensive knowledge of a wide diversity of differing value systems. However, they are unable to comparatively evaluate these systems without appealing to mediating values that must themselves be justified by other mediating values—and so on down the justificatory line until we have an undefended assertion or an infinite regress.[11] Bedrock values, then, do not come from philosophers. In democracies, they are the domain of communities and publics.

EVIDENCE CLASSIFICATION SCHEME

To better estimate where experts can be helpful, to help experts produce clearer and better guidelines, and to sort out expert guidance effectively, it would help to be explicit about the fact and value claims that undergird experts' recommendations. This objective would be facilitated by the employment of a simple evidence classification scheme (ECS). The ECS would evaluate diagnostic, treatment, and emergency response guidelines, and other specific action guides, by rating the doxastic security of the claims that constitute its fact and value components. The term *doxastic* refers to belief. When we inquire about the "doxastic security" of a claim, we are inquiring about the stability of the beliefs it explicitly manifests.

Recall that every guideline or action guide implicitly contains both fact and value claims. This amalgam suggests a four-type evidence classification scheme in which both factual claims (F claims) and value claims (V claims) are rated as either doxastically secure (firmly grounded, not highly susceptible to major revision or dispute) or doxastically vulnerable (not firmly grounded, likely to be revised or disputed). There will, of course, be borderline or intermediate cases where the classification as secure or vulnerable is itself disputed. However, adding an intermediate category would not help appreciably; it would just double the possible loci for debate. If claims are not secure, then we should regard them as vulnerable.

F claims are considered "firmly grounded" when they are backed by good supporting evidence. Sometimes the supporting evidence will be of the nature of formal scientific studies, but often these are not necessary. There is good supporting evidence for the belief that the sun will rise tomorrow, even apart from scientific studies. V claims, on the other hand, are grounded in moral convictions, preferences, and such—things that cannot be definitively mediated by scientific studies. Scientific studies can show the prevalence and distribution of various moral convictions and preferences (as in opinion polls and descriptive ethics research), and how the operation of one value may interfere with the fulfillment of others (as, for instance, in showing the economic effects of particular government policies). Ultimately, however, value claims must rest on convictions that cannot be definitively established through reason or empirical studies (a point discussed in chapter 3). From the standpoints of public policy and social ethics, V claims typically are considered doxastically secure when they reflect values that are widely shared in the target population.

The suggested ECS would beget four types of action guide:

— Type I Guides (Generally Secure): F claims secure, V claims secure
— Type II Guides (Factually Vulnerable): F claims vulnerable, V claims secure
— Type III Guides (Normatively Vulnerable): F claims secure, V claims vulnerable
— Type IV Guides (Generally Vulnerable): F claims vulnerable, V claims vulnerable

The following (from an article on smallpox as a biological weapon) is an example of a Type I (generally secure) action guide: "The discovery of a single suspected case of smallpox must be treated as an international health emergency and be brought immediately to the attention of national officials through local and state health authorities."[12] Of note, this and similar action guides have formed the basis for coercive reporting requirements that have been widely accepted with little controversy.[13] The primary F claims for this action guide include the propositions that (1) smallpox is a serious illness, (2) smallpox is transmissible, (3) there is a large population of persons who are potentially vulnerable to smallpox infection, (4) health officials' knowledge of new cases of smallpox would lead to preventive actions, and (5) some of these preventive actions (for instance, immunization of contacts or likely contacts) could save many lives. Each of these claims is well warranted empirically. The primary V claim is that saving many lives by preventing smallpox infections is good and worth doing, even in the face of possible negative consequences such as immunization reactions, excessive worry, and various forms of clinical and social overreaction. This claim is also unlikely to be seriously disputed.

The somewhat infamous plastic taping tactic is a Type II (factually vulnerable) action guide pertaining to civilian bioterror response. It has appeared in multiple sources, most notably in Senator Bill Frist's (otherwise mostly helpful) book on what ordinary citizens need to know about bioterrorism. Frist advises that people who find themselves indoors in a situation where biological or chemical weapons may have been deployed outside should close their vents and then "seal windows and doors with plastic tape."[14] The primary F claim is that ordinary citizens who suspect that chemical or biological weapons have been deployed outside will be safer and perhaps also more sanguine if they seal themselves off from the external environment. This controversial claim may well be true, but it is not solidly supported by evidence.[15] Thus far, the approach has apparently led (through misapplication) to two deaths, while producing no documented saves.[16] Hence, the F claim is doxastically vulnerable. The V claims behind this guideline, on the other hand, are straightforward. Self-preservation is a widely acknowledged value, and virtually everyone agrees that it is worth the expense of a roll of plastic tape.

In a Type III (normatively vulnerable) action guide, the F claim is doxastically secure, but here the V claim is vulnerable. An example is the recommendation by the Advisory Committee on Immunization Practices (ACIP) that the government withhold smallpox vaccine from U.S. citizens who desire to obtain it.[17] The factual claims behind this action guide are widely accepted and include claims that (1) the likelihood of a smallpox attack is uncertain but small, (2) smallpox vaccine is relatively dangerous in comparison to other vaccines, (3) smallpox vaccine poses risks not just for vacinees themselves but also for their contacts, (4) the understanding of medical risks and benefits of vaccines is not good among typical members of the general public in the United States, and (5) in the event of a smallpox outbreak, exposed parties have up to 72 hours to be vaccinated without sacrificing benefits. One possible factual point of contention concerns the likelihood that public health officials could deliver the vaccine quickly enough to exposed parties. This point does not, however, appear to be pivotal to the ACIP recommendations. The value claims are another matter. As Thomas May and Ross D. Silverman detail in a nicely done article on smallpox vaccination for the general public, dissenting parties bring cogent objections to the ACIP strategy on ethical grounds that informed citizens should be at liberty to obtain vaccinations when the primary danger is to themselves.[18] Though May and Silverman ultimately come down on the side of the ACIP recommendations, they make it clear that this is a difficult ethical issue.

The final category is the Type IV (generally vulnerable) action guide, where both fact and value claims are open to serious dispute. This sort of action guide is distressingly common in coercive guidelines for mass casualty medicine for several reasons. First (regarding F claims), research in disaster medicine is in its infancy (at least relative to many other domains of biomedical research). Second (also regarding F claims), the infrequency and diversity of serious disasters poses significant barriers to prospective disaster studies and to meta-analyses of studies from different disasters, and the lethality of many chemical and bioterror agents precludes clinical trials. Third (regarding V claims), the values that justify coercion are in tension with several countervailing ethical values, making coercion an inherently contentious issue. Fourth (also regarding V claims), the primary value that justifies coercion—security—is weighed in highly divergent ways by different persons and different moral communities. Typically, security overrides liberty only when threshold levels of danger or risk are involved. Specifying these thresholds is difficult.

Marcia Welby's recommendation to quarantine her tularemia patient in chapter 1 is based on a Type IV action guide. It contains an explicit F claim that the patient poses a significant transmission risk to her infant, and an implicit V claim that saving lives is more important than respecting informed patient decisions. Both are highly susceptible to counterargument.

It is important to recognize that type IV action guides are not the equivalent of bad or low-quality advice. To the contrary, their major feature is merely that they are disputable on both factual and ethical terms. Often some action is necessary, and they are the best that we can do. Depending on the cogency of the disputed claims, type IV guides can be high-quality or low-quality. A high-quality type IV guideline would presumably contain an explanation of where it came from (i.e., the reasons, opinions, precedents and other input on which it is based) as well as an admission of its doxastic vulnerability.

It is also important to understand that doxastic security is a far cry from invincibility. That means that even type I guides are fallible. New evidence may bring previously sturdy F claims into doubt. Cultural changes may erode V claims. To be doxastically secure is to enjoy a relatively stable and privileged position in the hierarchy of collective beliefs. This privilege evolves, in the case of F claims, largely (or at least ideally) from scientific evidence and collective experience. Its genesis in the case of V claims is various and somewhat disputed, but its manifestations are clearly in mutual habits of thought and judgment.

Sometimes different parties will offer diverging reasons for the same proposed action. One party may offer good reasons, while another party offers poor ones. And sometimes parties will agree on most of the facts but will slant them differently based on value considerations. Both possibilities seem to have applied in the debate about the National Quarantine Act of 1893, which ostensibly hinged on the factual issue of whether or not immigrants were a major source of infectious outbreaks of typhoid and cholera in New York City. Underlying the F claims was a dispute between proponents of germ theory and anti-contagionists. From the vantage point of contemporary hindsight, the germ theorists offered better reasons. Yet interestingly, germ theorists (like the anti-contagionists) came down on both sides of the issue. Highly respected T. Mitchell Prudden, M.D., championed the view that harsh immigration restrictions were not necessary to control infectious outbreaks of cholera. An even more prominent physician, William Osler, M.D., joined physicians from Johns Hopkins University who cited cholera risks in petitioning the president to suspend all immigration. Both were germ theorists, and both made F claims that would be cogent even today. As Howard Markel argues, it was more often a value question that carried the day—would Americans be morally and materially better off without so many immigrants?[19] Prudden's and Osler's guidance is type IV, bordering on type III (save for an ostensible disagreement about the likelihood that alternative measures, besides immigration restriction, could better avert the epidemic).

The proposed evidence classification scheme is easier to apply and likely to be most useful in reference to focused action guides. Very general action guides such as the National Response Plan or the Model State Emergency Health Powers Act contain a broad array of smaller action guides that are better rated individually than as a whole.

One of the major benefits of an ECS is that it helps us sort out where scientific experts are helpful and where their advice is essentially irrelevant. Type I (generally secure) guides are uncontroversial, yet their formulation often requires input from experts who can explain and apply advanced technical knowledge.

Type II (factually vulnerable) guides hinge on factual issues. Hence, application of the highest possible standards of evidence is crucial. Methodological expertise (particularly in methods of interpreting data) sometimes becomes the most important factor in sorting out possible options. Convening consensus panels of "expert" practitioners and researchers is a popular way of navigating factual dilemmas and might seem appropriate in the formulation of type II action guides. However, accomplished practitioners often lack methodological skills, and medical researchers are typically more adept at designing studies than at interpreting them objectively.[20] Finding the right experts can be a challenge.

Type III (normatively vulnerable) guides hinge on value issues and thus fall into the public domain. In the debate over a Type III action guide, experts may be useful for clarifying fact-related matters such as probability computations, but their specific recommendations carry no particular weight (contrary to the deference that many government officials have shown toward the ACIP recommendations on voluntary mass immunization).

Type IV (generally vulnerable) action guides typically require input both from experts and from the general public, but here, as wherever V claims are vulnerable, the greatest liability is that participation by the general public will be insufficient. The tendency to assume the priority of good reasons legitimacy over public justification legitimacy (discussed in chapter 3) and to mistake value claims for fact claims may lead to overreliance on scientific experts in formulating such action guides.

In sum, scientific expertise tends to be the most important quality for agents formulating Type I and Type II action guides. In Type III guides it is adjunctive at best. And in Type IV action guides, scientific expertise is of variable importance but always requires supplementation from publicly accountable deliberators.

Because experts and the public have a basic intuitive awareness of these utilities, scientific experts who seek political or economic influence often seek to portray Type III and IV action guides as Type I or II guides. One common way to pull this off, especially in public health circles, is to pretend that controversial or undecided ethical issues—the meaning of social justice, for instance—have been essentially resolved. Another strategy is to reframe factual issues in terms that usurp ethical issues or transform the ethical issues into something relatively superfluous. LILCO's evacuation plan attempts both transformation and usurpation. The plan should be regarded as a Type IV action guide (even though it would be better to apply ECS to its individual components). It contains a disputable F claim that inhabitants could be evacuated in cars and buses quickly enough so that they would not be at significant risk. It contains a disputable V claim that attendant radiation risks, in the event of a meltdown, are ethically acceptable. LILCO's experts tried to portray their plan as a Type I action guide by (1) shifting the risk-benefit analysis for the proposed reactor in the direction of benefits by overstating the likelihood of successful evacuation (thus transforming a difficult value-balancing problem into a relatively trivial one); and (2) conflating statistical risk analysis with the ethical assessment of risks (thus usurping the ethical problem by implying that acceptable risk is a scientific issue). The latter species of subterfuge also seems to have been propounded (perhaps more successfully, though the final verdict is not yet in) by the ACIP panel. A risk-benefit analysis can be infinitely thoughtful, elaborate, meticulous, and informed; but it can never be legitimately converted, by scientific experts alone, into a guideline for public action. There is simply no objectively verified formula for determining the proper equilibrium between dueling values.

Another benefit of the ECS is that it helps us distinguish between solid, evidence-based practices and practices that are based merely on reasonable projections. This knowledge should aid policy makers and other deliberators; and by highlighting areas where evidence is lacking, it will help us to formulate a defensible research agenda.

NEWS AND ENTERTAINMENT MEDIA AS INFORMATION MEDIATORS

News and entertainment media exert powerful effects on public deliberation about MCM by informing public perceptions of risk, collective behavior, preparedness, and the need for coercion. Often they are the primary lens through which policy makers and the public are exposed to scientific data pertaining to disasters.[21] Sometimes they relay information in a relatively direct manner, such as in newspaper articles and news reports. Often, however, information is relayed implicitly and subtly—as in editorial allusions or fictional tales. In both cases, accuracy and reliability may be suspect.

In direct reporting, the information-relaying function can be compromised by reporters' relative scientific ignorance or by the tendency to focus on "good stories" and to slant reporting to enhance dramatic appeal.[22] News media and fictional media both tend to reinforce disaster myths—which eventually take on the character of dogma, even with government policy makers and professional disaster planners.[23] Though these pitfalls are often attributed to media sensationalism and prejudice, other less direct sources also pertain. For instance, news media understandably turn to the quickest, most obvious, most available sources for a breaking story. This tendency has caused them to focus on command sources in disaster reporting—often neglecting or missing ad hoc action by victims, bystanders, and volunteers (despite their potential newsworthiness) and framing disasters from the standpoint of government officials.[24]

Movies, television shows, and novels that deal with bioterrorism, epidemics, chemical warfare, and other MCM-related themes are typically replete with reinforcement for erroneous dogmas such as beliefs that ordinary people usually panic in disasters or upon learning they are in imminent danger, that looting and lawlessness prevail when social restraints and law enforcement capacities are compromised by disaster, that many people experiencing disasters are stunned to the point of prolonged incapacity, and that a strong central command is the key to managing disasters successfully. Each of these claims has been contradicted by voluminous research evidence.[25] And *each of these false dogmas tends to augment preconceptions that coercion is necessary in the management of disasters.*

The social disorder in New Orleans after Hurricane Katrina is an illustrative case. Katrina was exceptional for a disaster in that significant looting and lawlessness occurred (the latter probably being related to the extent of social disruption—Katrina should be classified as a "catastrophe" rather than as an ordinary disaster). Yet it was typical in that disaster relief efforts were hampered far more by inaccurate reports of lawlessness than by the actual occurrence of lawlessness.[26] In the days following the hurricane, there were reports that the city had been virtually overrun by roving bands of thugs who raped, killed, and pillaged. As the *New York Times* later reported: "The fears changed troop deployments, delayed medical evacuations, drove police officers to quit, grounded helicopters. Edwin P. Compass III, the police superintendent, said that tourists—the core of the city's economy—were being robbed and raped on streets that had slid into anarchy."[27] Other effects of the perception of lawlessness included coercive measures such as forced evacuation and firearm confiscation (the latter apparently applied only to law-abiding citizens—on the mystifying premise that they would be less vulnerable to armed thugs if they were themselves unarmed). Yet as things settled down a few weeks later, officials could document not a single murder, and no one reported being raped. Looting had occurred (sometimes with an aim to meeting survival needs, sometimes simply for material gain), but at nothing close to the originally reported magnitude. In other words, disaster relief efforts were derailed by a proliferation of rumors. These rumors did not originate with the news media, but the media certainly seized upon them—and transmitted them ad nauseam.

Should society hold news and entertainment to standards of accuracy and veracity in portraying and reporting disasters? A careful consideration of this question runs afield of this book's focus. Certainly legal sanctions for poorly grounded reporting hardly seem in order (this rationale might be extended, after all, to the academy). Perhaps pressure for better media performance could be exerted by an informed public—for instance, by predicating patronage on a reputation for veracity and thoroughness. More realistically, I believe the press would respond if self-proclaimed disaster experts quit giving them inaccurate information. The panic and looting myths, for instance, are widely embraced among government officials dealing with disasters and appear frequently in their statements and guidelines.[28] Media cannot be blamed for believing them.

A simple evidence classification scheme would also help immensely in this regard. Media should routinely query experts about the evidence for guidelines and predictions. From the standpoint of public policy, the media should be viewed as an essential adjunct to disaster preparedness and (as we will later discuss) response. They will either help or they will hinder. But in virtually every case, they will play a crucial role.

CHAPTER FIVE

Public Deliberation and Strategic Leadership

Politically legitimate decisions about the use of coercion require not only the right kind of deliberation but also deliberation by the right people. Simply designating an amorphous "public" will hardly do. Where coercion is considered, it is important to determine who should have a right to input, where the authority for a final decision should lie, and what sorts of constraints should apply to this authority. Without question, these items will vary in different contexts.

The most obvious qualification for a right to deliberative input is the likelihood that one will be affected by a proposed intervention. In clinical and organizational ethics, affected parties are often referred to as "stakeholders" and their interests (or "stakes") in a given clinical decision are characterized, then roughly compared and contrasted. Decisional input from deeply affected parties generally carries more weight than input from those who are affected only peripherally. That is why, for instance, input from competent patients is accorded such a high priority—they are usually the ones most profoundly affected by medical interventions.

A similar weighing of interests usually pertains in public health ethics and public policy. Just as medicine recognizes a principle of the autonomy of individual patients for medical treatment decisions, public health (sometimes) recognizes a principle of weighted autonomy of individuals, communities, and populations for decisions that affect their lives in a relatively exclusive way.

Unfortunately, strong strains of paternalism also exist in public health practice. The recent attack on medical paternalism mounted by bioethicists and other scholarly critics never really extended into the territory of public health. Thus, public health officials painlessly lapse into thinking that health is an invariant universal value that is precisely understood only by experts, and that health promotion is such a serious, difficult, and complicated task that it should be closely overseen and controlled by experts such as themselves. I hope that the preceding chapters have dispatched this view.

Our first concern now is to determine how stakeholders should be identified for participation in public deliberative processes in which coercion is proposed, a problem that frequently hinges on two types of concern: how interests should be weighted, and how deliberative bodies can be limited to workable sizes. These factors play out differently depending on the scope of anticipated effects, the simplest case being decisions for individual action that primarily affect the actor.

RIGHT DELIBERATORS FOR SELF-REGARDING DECISIONS

The first, most obvious, and in many cases most compelling source of interest in coercive decisions is the interest inhering in those who will be objects of coercion. As we have observed, individuals typically have a strong prima facie interest in not being forced to surrender their autonomy. In clinical medicine, the prerogative for self-governance begets a virtually inviolable right of competent patients not to be touched or restrained against their will. Two sorts of general ethical criteria exist for abridging this liberty: (1) the patient is unable to make an informed decision (usually due either to impaired decisional capacity or to time constraints that preclude informed decision making), or (2) the result of not restraining the patient would probably be serious harm to the public's health. Thus, we take seriously injured comatose patients to the operating room without their permission; and patients with certain infectious conditions (e.g., tuberculosis) are sometimes required to undergo directly observed treatment. As we will shortly observe, both of these general ethical criteria apply (albeit differently) in public health decisions about coercion.

If we extend principles of clinical ethics to public health practice, we would rule out the prevention of self-harm (PSH) as a general rationale for coercive public health interventions—except where something like the two aforementioned abridgement criteria pertained (the second criterion actually hinges on PHO, the prevention of harm to others). Motorcycle helmet laws were earlier cited as an example of a public health intervention based on PSH. Both inadequate decisional capacity (motorcyclists not having the sophistication to understand risks) and harm to the public (covering bikers' medical treatment) have been proposed as rationale for such laws; but (as we observed) these strained arguments function mostly as a cover for dismissive judgments about bikers' conceptions of the good life. Seatbelt laws are a better example of justifiable legislation based on PSH. The harm to the public by way of medical bills is certainly much greater with non-seatbelt-use than with non-motorcycle-helmet-use. More importantly, there are better reasons for holding that non-seatbelt-use rarely manifests an informed decision. Persons get into the habit of not wearing seatbelts and are dulled to the risks through uneventful repetition. Typically, not wearing a seatbelt expresses no opinion about the good life, or even a conscious decision. Rather, it manifests a maladaptive habit. Maladaptive habits are, of course, inadequate decisional devices. People need help breaking this habit, and coercive seatbelt laws—so the argument goes—are the most workable solution.

From the philosopher's armchair, coercion seems a drastic way to reverse such bad habits. Education is of course much preferable—when it works. But people do not usually respond to risk reduction strategies when the risks do not concern them. It is a great irony of public safety that citizens will clamor for access to gas masks, smallpox vaccinations, and home antibiotic reserves to protect themselves against extremely remote terrorist threats; but they will not take the simplest precautions against prevalent hazards that consistently kill large numbers of people.

This brings us to prevention of self-harm as a rationale for coercion in mass casualty medicine. For the most part, it is unreasonable to presume that PSH legislation will be necessary to disrupt bad habits resulting from unconcern about nuclear, biological, and chemical threats. People tend, if anything, to be overly concerned about these things. When PSH is applied in MCM, it will probably be either (1) to prevent agents from choosing dangerous and unnecessary self-protective actions, or (2) to prevent self-harm where time constraints preclude informed decision making.[1] Both of these objectives are based on concern that citizens will not be able to make informed decisions.

The first objective pertains when threats of force are used to prevent ordinary citizens from obtaining smallpox immunizations (a policy analogous to prescription laws). May and Silverman cautiously support this policy for the following reasons: (1) citizens lack relevant information that would be necessary to make an informed choice because the new (Baxter International and Acambis) smallpox vaccine is experimental in nature and may have unanticipated side effects even after FDA approval; (2) citizens typically have difficulty acting rationally when exposed to terrifying but vague threats such as that of smallpox; (3) the smallpox vaccine is a relatively dangerous one, and adverse reactions to this vaccine might undermine public confidence in other more important and less dangerous vaccines; and (4) the smallpox vaccine is a live-virus vaccine that can cause harm to the contacts of vaccinated persons. May and Silverman emphasize the fourth point—arguing in essence that preventing access to voluntary immunization is not based solely on PSH.

Each of these considerations constitutes a mini-argument. Cumulatively, they seem to May and Silverman to justify the infringement of liberty that occurs when bans on voluntary public immunization are enforced. But I think May and Silverman set the scales too far in the direction of security. Their action guide is Type IV, and it is questionable on several fronts.

The first mini-argument is that citizens should not have access to the smallpox vaccine because its risks are uncertain. This type of argument is common in many contexts (especially investigational drug regulations). Despite its prevalence, the argument is a poor one. It is based on a highly contentious, even ridiculous, V claim—that it is impossible to make an informed affirmative choice when risks are uncertain. But informed consent requires a grasp of relevant and available information, not—as this argument presumes—that a particular threshold quantity of information must be available. From this initial contestable V claim comes another doubly contestable V claim—that government should not allow people to take nonquantifiable risks. The unevenness with which this spurious norm is applied in contemporary American society is stunning. Mountaineers are free to attempt highly dangerous first ascents (where the unpredictability of weather and the uncharted terrain make the risk very uncertain), and we glorify them when they do. But women dying of ovarian cancer are prevented from access to promising experimental drugs until the FDA can attest that they are effective and safe.

The second mini-argument contends (with ample documentation) that people contemplating terrifying exotic threats such as smallpox tend to make skewed risk-benefit assessments. This consideration is relevant. One fact that it does not account for, however, is the benefit that accrues from having fears—even overwrought fears—assuaged. Moreover, it is impossible for the government or any other secular authority to state precisely what counts as a cogent risk-benefit analysis, since risks and benefits depend on conceptions of the good—conceptions that democratic, pluralistic polities allow citizens to form for themselves. This prerogative should be rescinded only when threats are particularly grave and ubiquitously acknowledged, and when circumstances preclude effective individual deliberation. The likely threat from smallpox vaccine hardly qualifies. Previous smallpox vaccines killed between one and two in a million. Even if the new vaccine killed three per million, we would lose less than eight hundred people if all non-immune-compromised people in the United States were immunized (meanwhile gaining national immunity against smallpox). And that would be a one-time-only affair. We lose as many every year traveling back and forth for the Fourth of July holiday. Perhaps we'd be better off if we cancelled one extended weekend and let people get immunized.

The third mini-argument against voluntary smallpox immunization—that adverse reactions to the smallpox vaccine would undermine public confidence in vaccines—hardly rates comment. In essence, this argument has us coerce people to gain their trust—a bad general strategy, and especially bad in this context. Should smallpox vaccine become available to the general public, explicit warnings that it is a relatively dangerous vaccine would be required of any clinician administering the vaccine; and the government could reinforce these warnings with various forms of public education. True, the media would undoubtedly attend fervently to serious adverse reactions, perhaps causing elements of the public to regard the vaccine as even more risky than it actually is. But if that were the case, then other mini-arguments holding that people overestimate the risk-benefit profile in favor of immunization would no longer hold. Meanwhile, should an actual terrorist attack with smallpox occur, wariness about the vaccine would hardly prevent people from taking action to protect themselves against the virus.

The fourth mini-argument invokes the second general ethical criterion for limiting personal liberty in self-regarding decisions—that the proposed actions in reality may cause significant public harm. That is, potential harm from smallpox vaccine is not entirely self-limited, since contacts may be harmed as well. This consideration might carry the day if harm to contacts was serious and common. Probably it warrants withholding the vaccine from individuals with immune-compromised family members. However, the incidence of serious harm to contacts is so miniscule that it cannot be meaningfully computed. If we start using such small effects as a means for denying individuals the prerogative to make their own risk-benefit analyses, the allowed scope of personal autonomy will be severely contracted.

Personally, I think that the likelihood of a smallpox attack on America is very small, and I have no inclination whatsoever to get immunized for it. That many others agree is attested by the lack of participation in the federal smallpox vaccine program for designated clinical providers. This pallid response seems to belie predictions that people will flock en masse to the clinics if voluntary smallpox immunization is allowed. In any case, my personal assessment of the risks and benefits of smallpox immunization, like those of my colleagues, is based largely on values and worldview impressions that I cannot fully justify before a pluralistic public. If we allow voluntary immunization—presumably with a strong official stance that it is not advised—public trust in government will be enhanced, not undermined. If there is a clear message from such a policy, it is that citizens should take part in deliberation about terrorism and mass casualty medicine. Such a policy would lead to greater public knowledge about smallpox.

The second objective justifying infringement of self-regarding decisional rights in MCM is to prevent self-harm where time constraints preclude informed decision making. This infringement proviso is called "emergency privilege," and it is well-described in the clinical literature. When safety hinges on immediate action, prolonged deliberation is folly. Rather, the most informed and knowledgeable persons—if there is a subgroup that clearly fits this description—should have temporary decisional authority.

Suppose, for example, a small bomb explodes near the center of a crowded football stadium. No one is hurt in the blast, but a pale yellow vapor is released, forming a cloud that drifts northward out of the stadium with the prevailing winds. Though many people come in contact with the vapor, most are free of symptoms. A large security force is already present, and they are instructed by emergency management leaders to secure a large area south of the stadium for decontamination. Though positive identification of the vapor is pending, authorities strongly suspect it contained a vesicant such as sulfur mustard or nitrogen mustard. Unlike Lewisite, nerve agents, and choking agents, mustards cause delayed blistering and airway difficulties that can be very serious or even fatal. These signs usually develop over two to twenty-four hours. The only way to prevent them is with thorough decontamination—best accomplished with total disrobing, followed by copious water irrigation (just a little water could spread the vesicant over the body without removing it).

After an initial disorganized quick-shuffle toward the exits, the crowd calms quickly. No one seems to be ill or hurt, and some fans even grumble that the authorities have overreacted by stopping the game. Voices over the loudspeaker announce that an attack with vesicants or other chemical agents is suspected and that everyone should make their way through the south exits, quickly disrobe, and proceed through the ladder-pipe mass decontamination system that the fire department has hastily constructed. Rescuers and police in protective gear arrive to assist. For the most part, people are cooperative, but two sorts of objection begin to crop up among segments of the crowd: (1) Some people say they are fine and insist on leaving. These individuals tend to become angry when police prevent them from leaving the warm zone (i.e., a relatively safe but somewhat contaminated area where casualties await or undergo decontamination). (2) Some people refuse to completely disrobe, saying they'll opt for death over public nudity.

I suggest that this is a situation in which coercion based on PSH may be legitimate and necessary. The relevant facts are as follows: (1) there is good reason to believe that many persons in the stadium have been exposed to dangerous or lethal concentrations of mustard agents; (2) it is impossible to tell on clinical grounds which persons are dangerously exposed; (3) though patients are 90 percent decontaminated if they quickly and completely disrobe, mustard agents require especially copious irrigation for complete decontamination (which is the only workable treatment);

(4) it is essential that this irrigation be accomplished quickly to prevent morbidity; (5) because persons are currently without symptoms, some are unimpressed with the danger and will not cooperate or listen attentively; and (6) if noncooperators were released from the warm zone without decontamination, they would *not* pose a serious health threat to others (even though they would contaminate other people and things, causing minor afflictions). In view of items (1) and (6), we can say that decisions not to undergo decontamination are primarily self-harming.

Two coercive options present themselves, both based on PSH. First, we could detain objecting parties until they agree to undergo decontamination. Second, we could decontaminate objecting parties by force. The first option is less coercive and gives noncooperating individuals time to rethink matters. Ideally, workers could be assigned to answer their questions and give more information. The pitfall is that precious time would be wasted, and if such patients wait until they develop symptoms, they are likely to develop serious medical problems. The second option overcomes this pitfall, but at the cost of extreme coercion. Forced disrobing and irrigation is analogous in some respects to rape, and might produce serious psychological trauma for some victims. Such harms are simply too great, I believe, for this option to be considered in any but the most exotic and unusual instances.

With both options, certain mitigating actions are possible. Personal decontamination kits (to be discussed in the next chapter) provide a means of protecting privacy during and after disrobing. Rescuers could also provide the alternative of a corridor decontamination system (which allows relative privacy) for patients who insist on modesty. These patients might have to wait longer for decontamination, but that is better than not decontaminating them and better than disrobing them by force. In the end, it will be the spirit of accommodation—not the willingness to coerce—that is most likely to carry the day successfully.

To summarize, the right deliberator for a self-regarding decision is the self who is affected. Advisors can be helpful, but others should not usurp the individual's autonomy in such instances unless: (1) the individual is seriously hampered (either by personal limitations or by time constraints) in the ability to understand or process relevant information; or (2) potentially harmful effects on others are significant enough to rescind the decision's "self-regarding" status.

RIGHT DELIBERATORS FOR FAR-REACHING DECISIONS

Unfortunately, establishing a noncoercion policy for self-regarding actions doesn't settle very much. Most of the proposed uses of coercion in MCM pertain to decisions and actions that cannot fairly be construed as self-regarding. Isolation and quarantine, for instance, is justified on the basis that infected parties are contagious and can seriously harm many others. And the conscription of health care providers is justified on the basis of far-reaching benefits they can provide in a public health emergency.

In such cases, some form of public deliberation is necessary—either advance deliberation that sets a policy to be implemented by officials, or situational deliberation that decides a particular issue (ideally there will be both). The earlier questions about how to weigh competing interests in choosing deliberators, how to keep the number of deliberators manageable, and how to structure authority for final decisions all present difficult challenges. These are foundational issues for deliberative democracy. Because it is beyond our scope to examine them in great detail, we will begin with a few simplifying general assumptions.

First, we will assume that it is possible to obtain valid deliberative input from a local community (understood geographically) or moral community (understood ideologically[2]), once the geographic or ideological boundaries are settled. What constitutes "valid" input will not be debated here beyond what has already been said— that in valid deliberation, the objective is a modus vivendi acceptable to each major deliberator or deliberative group. It is easier to define the boundaries (i.e., criteria of inclusion and exclusion) for a local community than for a moral community. On the other hand, it is easier to construct internally valid decisional criteria for a moral community than for a local community (since the problem of ethical pluralism is mitigated). One of the problems with using moral communities as deliberative bodies is that citizens cannot easily be classified on the basis of membership in such communities—the majority of citizens in pluralistic democracies have mixed allegiances to somewhat incompatible moral communities. And some citizens seem to have few permanent allegiances.[3] Another problem with using moral communities is that deliberation within a group (generally regarded as a prelude to sending representatives to higher-level intergroup deliberations) tends to magnify the differences that distinguish it from other groups.[4]

In line with these considerations, the second assumption is that the primary boundary-forming functions in mass casualty medicine are geographic in nature and that smaller geographic units can find a way to fairly navigate ethical pluralism. This assumption follows most of the theoretical work on deliberative democracy, which assumes local community as the context. Devices such as deliberative polling and a special "deliberation day" have been proposed to elicit balanced and thoughtful input from citizens with diverse moral visions.[5] These devices are particularly relevant to the formulation of MCM policies, since mass casualty events afflict particular geographic communities, generally without focusing on particular moral communities. In most mass casualty events, the particular afflicted geographic community is inevitably the primary responder. In the face of such tragedies—and in planning for them—requirements for cooperation preclude the usual degree of mutual indifference between moral communities. Sometimes insularity is not an affordable luxury.

Decisions about coercion in mass casualty medicine can be roughly classified into four categories, carved in accordance with the immediacy and proximity of the problems they address: (1) policy decisions, (2) strategic leadership decisions, (3) tactical leadership decisions, and (4) decisions for individual action. Policy decisions typically occur in pre-event planning and optimally result from political processes that involve extensive public deliberation. An example is the passage of a state emergency health powers act such as the Delaware act discussed in an earlier chapter.

Strategic leadership decisions often involve the implementation of policy at the highest levels of leadership in situations that do not allow for extensive public deliberation or political wrangling. Suppose, for instance, there is an actual bioterrorism incident involving smallpox. A governor declaring a state quarantine or a public health authority setting up a mandatory smallpox vaccination program are examples of strategic leadership decisions that might follow.

Tactical leadership decisions are more focused on specific problems occurring at the front lines in a mass casualty event. An incident commander who decides to deploy a group of volunteers to a specific area for search and rescue activities is making a tactical leadership decision.

Decisions for particular actions are the most immediate and personal. Examples would include a physician triaging a patient, a rescuer asking a victim to disrobe and stand in line for ladder-pipe decontamination, or a police officer deciding to forcefully detain an unruly victim.

As with most useful classification schemes, the categories in this decisional taxonomy are not altogether discreet. That is, some decisions will be difficult to categorize because they lie at the border between two categories. Deciding to take control of a hotel for chemical casualty staging and decontamination is an example—it seems somewhere between strategic and tactical leadership decisions.

FEDERAL, STATE, AND LOCAL AUTHORITY

Jurisdictional disputes tend to erupt at each of the aforementioned decisional levels. At the policy and strategic leadership levels, for instance, there is a particularly prominent and longstanding dispute pitting federal versus state and/or local authorities. State and local rights controversies are, of course, as old as the republic; but in public health, disputation of this variety came to a head during the yellow fever, cholera, and smallpox epidemics of the nineteenth century. To a large extent, these epidemics (especially yellow fever) precipitated the movement toward a national public health authority in this country.

For roughly a century after the ratification of the Constitution, public health functions including quarantine fell primarily under state and local purview. Many nineteenth-century sanitationists and other public health advocates deplored this situation and succeeded in drawing attention to the abysmal performance of state and local authorities in containing yellow fever and other epidemics.[6] These advocates offered an alternative national public health model that was attractive on several fronts. First, it removed responsibility for public health decisions and practices from the hands of local officials who were beholden to local businesses. For these businesses (and for public officials who deferred to them), public health was typically less important than financial profit. Second, it offered the prospect of uniform standards for sanitation and quarantine — standards that may have lacked a firm evidentiary basis but had the virtue of according with the latest thinking about disease prevention.[7] Third, it portended a degree of uniformity in public health practices. This development would help immensely with data collection (thus mitigating the aforementioned problem with evidentiary basis), and it would also presumably facilitate communication between authorities from different jurisdictions. Fourth, the nationalization of public health would result in a consolidation of resources for use in public health enterprises, especially quarantine and epidemic control.

In 1878 the national sanitationists won a significant battle against states' rights advocates and moderate federalists (i.e., those who agreed that there should be a central public health authority but who believed it should contain representatives from the states) by securing a national quarantine board. Their National Board of Health didn't last very long (yellow fever dissipated and so did public concern), but by 1893 the cholera scare elevated an older, rival organization, the Marine Hospital Service, to prominence as a national public health agency.[8] Since then, national public health has traveled an uneven, adversarial, but in the end relentless, path to power.

Not that controversy has been laid to rest. As the magnitude of America's moral pluralism becomes more evident, and as state governments feel the sting of decreased federal funding, there has been a renaissance of states' rights rhetoric in American politics. This movement has penetrated the federal government and involved both major parties. Democrats, for instance, typically support state drug re-importation initiatives such as those championed by the state governments of Illinois and Maine. Republicans support state experiments in welfare and Medicaid, including the pioneering Oregon plan. In disaster medicine, Lawrence Gostin's emphasis on state planning and state powers has been endorsed by politicians from both parties. His group's Model State Emergency Health Powers Act (MSEHPA) has been favorably reviewed by a multitude of federal officials (usually without explicit endorsements), and it has influenced health powers legislation in a majority of states.

Those who emphasize state supremacy in mass casualty medicine point not only to the political legitimacy that pertains when local jurisdictions have a greater role in deciding their own policies and procedures, but also to several practical benefits of localized leadership. First and foremost, mass casualty events tend to occur abruptly, often with little warning, and typically require an immediate response if casualties are to be minimized. Given adequate planning and preparation, local systems are better situated than national systems to respond in a timely fashion. Second, most mass casualty events are geographically circumscribed. The commerce clause (the third paragraph of Section 8 of the U.S. Constitution) is frequently invoked as a rationale for federal involvement in evolving public health threats such as epidemics because these threats cross state boundaries and their proliferation can be tied to interstate commerce. However, most mass casualty events do not evolve or proliferate in the manner of epidemics. Chemical attacks will almost always be localized, and likewise with bombs, earthquakes, fires, and tornadoes. Hurricanes typically affect several states at once, but their damage patterns are not tied to commerce. There seems to be little constitutional basis for federal jurisdiction in such disasters—unless, of course, such is requested by the affected states. Third, many of the benefits of nationalized public health can be achieved, without depriving the states of jurisdiction, by employing federal agencies in advisory and supplemental roles. The MSEHPA is an obvious example of the advisory function. It was prepared under federal auspices and has been disseminated nationally, each state choosing elements that it finds salient. National standards and particular event-related guidance are provided by organizations such as the Centers for Disease Control and the Department of Energy—often without usurping legitimate forms of state sovereignty. The National Pharmaceutical Stockpile is managed by the CDC and provides an example of supplemental federal aid that is available in case state resources are overwhelmed.

Despite these considerations, contemporary national public health advocates still employ many of the considerations championed by nineteenth-century sanitationists (though details and priorities have changed). As we observed in an earlier chapter, national emergency management advocate George Annas adds another argument (one that would not have succeeded in the nineteenth century)—that national authorities should handle disaster response, since they are best equipped to do the job and they are the best guarantors of universal civil rights that get threatened during such a response. This addition is an important element of contemporary national public health advocacy, given the plausibility of states' rights rebuttals to earlier arguments.

Annas's perspective is an expression of liberal cosmopolitanism. He is, of course, more devoted than most liberal cosmopolitans to protecting individual prerogatives against government and corporate power. But this commitment is derailed by his willingness to canonize a robust array of moral absolutes—this array consisting largely of particular interpretations of constitutional rights (many of these being advertised as universal human rights) and political conventions articulated by an enclave of contemporary Western elites including Annas. For instance, Annas writes: "The model act seems to have been drafted for a different age; it is more appropriate for the United States of the 19th Century than for the United States of the 21st Century. Today, all adults have the constitutional right to refuse examination and treatment, and such a refusal should not result in involuntary confinement simply on the whim of a public health official. At the very least, persons suspected of having a contagious disease should have the option of being examined by physicians of their own choice and, if isolation is necessary, of being isolated in their own homes."[9]

This interpretation doesn't leave much room for genuine moral pluralism. Annas presumes that constitutional rights should be interpreted in fine detail by federal courts without latitude for local variation. When federal judges have strong moral intuitions, the law of the land and its mores should change to reflect them. Hence, Annas proclaims that "*today* all adults have a constitutional right" to refuse the sorts of interventions he finds suspect—as if the Constitution had actually been amended, subsequent to the nineteenth century, to express his view. This account contrasts sharply with that of states' rights (and modus vivendi) proponents such as John Calhoun and more moderate recent successors such as Louis Brandeis.[10]

In his commentary on the right to refuse medical interventions, Annas argues that involuntary confinement should not hinge "on the whim of a public health official" and that "persons suspected of having a contagious disease should have the option of being examined by physicians of their own choice" and of being isolated, if such is necessary, in their own homes. These seem (to me) to be sensible guidelines, but they come at a price and presume a specific account of the proper balance between liberty and security. Presumably, the opinion of public health officials about the need for isolation or quarantine will be more informed than that of ordinary citizens and perhaps more informed than the opinions of typical physicians. For (risk-averse) people in some localities, investing authority for such decisions in the hands of the latter may be regarded as taking an excessive risk. Furthermore, if we grant citizens a right to choose their own physicians, then efficiency may be severely compromised. And finally, at-home quarantine may be riskier in some jurisdictions than quarantine in facilities that can be easily monitored by public health officials. Though I would (and will) argue that Annas's suggestions are more sensible and less risky in typical U.S. jurisdictions than they seem to some critics, Annas's presumption that federal officials have legitimate authority to prescribe the liberty-security equilibrium in such detail is deeply problematic.

The centerpiece of Annas's argument against excessive coercion is the issue of trust. As I earlier observed, Annas thinks that: (1) trust is central to effective disaster response; (2) trust is undermined when coercion is employed unnecessarily; and (3) levels of trust are generally high, such that an uncoerced public can be expected to cooperate with most legitimate public health interventions. Annas is correct about each of these points. However, using trust to argue for restraint in coercion undermines his arguments for national control. In order to cultivate and protect trust, it is better to have local authorities in leadership positions.

Local leadership typically engenders more trust than federal leadership because: (1) local leaders are more apt to understand the nuance of local customs, mores, and practices; (2) local leaders are chosen by the local public; (3) local leaders are known more intimately by the local public; and (4) local leaders maintain role linkages that help optimize performance in mass casualty events. This last point may require a little explanation. By "role linkages" I refer to particular human relations or habits of cooperation that have a bearing on MCM activities. Under the heading of "role complementarity," researchers have recorded some of these relations and habits, and shown that they can enhance disaster response.[11] The list of possibly beneficial local role linkages is virtually endless and includes (briefly) linkages such as: city medical examiner with local physicians, fire officials with hotel managers, police with city government, EMS with fire department, emergency department directors with local public health officials, and city government with news media.

The best conclusion seems to be that authority in mass casualty medicine, including authority to enact coercive measures, should be as local as possible, given logistical realities and the range of threatened parties. When logistics allow, individuals should be able to make their own decisions about self-regarding behaviors. Likewise, local communities should have as much control as possible in managing events that are not apt to metastasize beyond their own boundaries. Federal personnel and resources are useful, depending on circumstances, in advisory and supportive capacities, but they should not have primary authority except where they are asked by state officials to assume this role or where federal intervention is needed to impede a serious and rapidly expanding threat that may cross state boundaries. These provisions are consistent with a relatively conservative reading of the commerce clause of the U.S. Constitution.

In planning for mass casualty events, the division of labor and authority between federal, state, and local officials should be delegated according to a sliding scale, depending on the nature of the anticipated hazards. Federal involvement and authority becomes incrementally more extensive as hazards exhibit characteristics such as rapid spreading (especially when state borders are being crossed), dangerousness to large numbers of persons, and intervention requirements that include technologically advanced and expensive measures or scarce resources that are best provided by federal sources.

One of the impediments to achieving intelligent, integrated, and effective jurisdictional assignments is the lack of a functional threat classification scheme. Currently, experts and policy makers tend to distinguish between three general types of mass casualty threat: (1) natural hazards (epidemics, earthquakes, hurricanes, tornadoes, floods); (2) accidental hazards (chemical spills, nuclear plant meltdown, explosions); and (3) attacks. Though much time and attention have lately been afforded to preparing for terrorist attacks, the immediate sources of damage due to attacks overlap with those of several natural and accidental hazards: biological attacks with epidemics, chemical attacks with chemical spills, radio-nuclear attacks with nuclear meltdowns, and conventional attacks with explosions. In some cases we have much more experience and data on accidental and natural hazards than on correlative attacks. An effective threat classification scheme, then, will employ categories that cross the boundaries between these various types of hazard.

This threat classification scheme will focus on strategic factors, especially (1) transmissibility (particularly between persons, though object-to-person or biological vector-to-person transmission may also be relevant); (2) magnitude and severity of likely harms; (3) duration (time interval) between event initiation and threat manifestation; and (4) duration of threat. These factors potentially have a major impact on appropriate levels of agency (e.g., federal vs. state) and on the justification for coercion. High transmissibility, especially, shifts the impetus toward higher levels of agency such as the federal government—a shift that is more pronounced when magnitude, severity, and duration are high. Shorter-duration threats are less amenable to help from afar and, for practical purposes, constitute an entirely different type of threat.

Some biological agents stand apart from nonbiological threats in being highly transmissible and liable to cause catastrophic international harm, and in posing a threat that could last years or even decades. Nuclear threats also can lay waste to large

TABLE 1
Biological-Chemical Agent Threat Classification

	L_1T_1	L_1T_2	L_2T_1	L_2T_2
D_1 Immediate	None	Saxitoxin Nerve Agents Phosgene Cyanide	None	Lewisite
D_2 Intermediate	None	Ricin Botulinum Tox Mustard Agents	None	SEB*
D_3 Long	Smallpox Hemorrhagic Fever Plague	Tularemia Anthrax	Shigellosis Cholera Influenza	VEE** Q Fever

*SEB = Staphylococcal Enterotoxin Type B
**VEE = Venezuelan Equine Encephalitis

areas for many years (though nuclear threats are easier to measure and contain).

Avian influenza has recently emerged as a global public health threat, though it is unlikely that it will be employed as a biological weapon. Among transmissible, deadly, and potentially global biological weapons threats, smallpox (*Variola major*), plague (*Yersinia pestis*), and hemorrhagic fevers are paramount. There are currently six "Category A" biological weapons agents, but only these three are highly transmissible from human to human—posing challenges that are very different than threats posed by the other "Category A" agents: *Bacillus anthracis* (anthrax), botulinum toxin, and *Francisella tularensis* (tularemia). Botulinum toxin is not a microorganism at all (it is a toxin produced by a microorganism), and its practical manifestations are more akin to a delayed-action chemical agent than to typical biological agents. Hence, smallpox, plague, and the hemorrhagic fevers require a special approach and should be regarded as a distinct threat category. To lump these agents together in a single category, as we now do,[12] invites confusion among rescuers, clinicians, and the public—a fact confronted regularly by those of us who have tried to impart information about biological terrorism.

As a step in the right direction, and as an example of the kind of practice-oriented classification scheme I have in mind, I propose a Biological-Chemical Agent Threat Classification (table 1) that employs three major categories. The first category is "duration prior to effects" (D). It expresses the length of the critical latency period that may exist between an attack or the initiation of an event and the development of clinical symptoms or other signs of damage.[13] D_1 denotes a duration of 0–1 hour (immediate). D_2 denotes a duration of 1–24 hours (intermediate). And D_3 denotes a duration greater than 24 hours (prolonged).

The second category is "lethality" (L). Here agents are classified as either "likely to be lethal" (L_1) or as "not likely to be lethal" (L_2). I consider an agent likely to be lethal if the mortality rate runs at 10 percent or higher. Even a relatively low mortality figure like 10 percent can cause mass dying when large numbers are affected.

The final category is "transmission" (T), which is divided into "likely" (T_1) and "not likely" (T_2).[14] Transmission is likely when the agent is known to have caused epidemics or to have the potential to cause epidemics. Though this criterion is less precise than the criteria in other categories, it is in practice easier to apply.

Outbreaks and attacks with the $D_3L_1T_1$ agents (smallpox, plague, hemorrhagic fevers, and possibly avian influenza) will always require a strong federal role. Hence, planning for such outbreaks should be organized, and to a large degree implemented, by federal authorities such as the CDC, FEMA, and the Department for Homeland Security (which now has higher-order authority over the former two). Oversight by Congress and the president are expected. And cooperation and integration with state and local authorities is, of course, crucial.

Outbreaks and attacks with $D_3L_2T_1$ agents (shigellosis, cholera, ordinary influenza) also pose a possible realm of jurisdiction for federal authorities, since they are transmissible and can cross state borders (and affect commerce). However, the need for federal oversight will vary from case to case. When local resources are sufficient, the federal role would presumably be small. Overall, this sort of agent does not constitute the most important threat and rarely falls under the domain of MCM. The best example, shigellosis, is minimally contagious and is significant primarily as a possible food-borne agent. Cholera is another possible $D_3L_2T_1$ agent, though the characteristics of this microbe vary significantly between strains. Cholera typically is waterborne. Influenza is much more highly transmissible than the other two, but thus far has not been regarded as a likely biological weapon.

The six other nonempty categories ($D_1L_1T_2$, $D_1L_2T_2$, $D_2L_1T_2$, $D_2L_2T_2$, $D_3L_1T_2$, $D_3L_2T_2$) should virtually always fall under local (or, at the highest, state) jurisdiction, with federal assistance as requested. Attacks with these agents garner brisk attention from national news media (e.g., sarin in 1985; anthrax in 2001; ricin in 2004); but the agents do not pose a threat of propagation, and, with the exception of anthrax, the most important ones produce only a brief and limited threat that is rapidly dispersed by nature. Federal intervention in most cases would be fruitless because the crucial interventions would need to occur almost immediately after awareness of the attacks. With anthrax, the most exceptional of these agents, federal assistance might be required (e.g., pharmaceutical stockpile for antibiotics if attack were large-scale, sophisticated laboratory and forensic technology). However, the need for assistance does not imply the resignation of jurisdiction.

The division of labor in policy making should reflect these distinctions. In strategic leadership, the distinctions (optimally) provide default boundaries—with room for negotiation in view of particular circumstances. Isolation and quarantine, for instance, are critically important coercive options that usually hinge on strategic leadership decisions by mayors, governors, public health authorities, or federal officials. Quarantine will in many cases be initiated at the local or state level—but cases that prompt it will virtually always involve dangerous transmissible agents that evoke a legitimate federal interest, ratified by the commerce clause. Emergency conscription also occurs at the strategic leadership level. This intervention could be local, state, or federal, depending on the magnitude of personnel needs. Each jurisdiction should be ready to make the critical decisions and to communicate with leaders at other levels of jurisdiction.

Once these jurisdictional boundaries are tentatively carved out, the most important elements of effective MCM and associated legitimate uses of coercion will be communication, cooperation, coordination, and continuity between the functioning agents—issues that will dominate the discussion as we consider questions of legitimate agency at the levels of tactical leadership and individual action.

CHAPTER SIX

Tactical Leadership

"Everyone's running up to first class. I've got to go. Bye."

After these final words to her husband, Sandy Bradshaw presumably joined the battle for United Airlines Flight 93. The cockpit voice recorder captured loud thumps, crashes, breaking glass, and shouting voices as passengers stormed past the fallen flight crew in an attempt to wrest control from their terrorist captors. Terrorists in the cockpit quickly realized they were losing the battle and were about to lose the plane. Twenty minutes short of their intended collision with the White House or Capitol Building, they intentionally crashed.[1]

United 93 fell in an empty field in Shanksville, Pennsylvania, at 10:03 a.m. on September 11, 2001. Through their improvised assault on the terrorist pilots, United 93 passengers probably saved the lives of hundreds of others, radically eclipsing any results obtained by officials tasked with overseeing their safety. It was the tactical highpoint of a very grim day.

There is much to learn from the battle for United 93, and perhaps even more to learn from our failures on 9/11. *The Final Report of the National Commission on Terrorist Attacks Upon the United States* (the 9/11 Commission Report) never focuses on the problem of justifying coercion in mass casualty medicine. Yet the report is an important source for our inquiry because it contains an unprecedented wealth of firsthand and proximate secondhand information about public leadership, tactics, adaptability, and human behavior in a dire public emergency.

SOME LESSONS FROM THE SEPTEMBER 11 AIRSPACE DEFENSE

As the 9/11 Commission Report amply demonstrates, the defense of U.S. airspace against the 9/11 terrorists was not achieved by executing protocols or by relying on a pre-established emergency chain of command. Rather, it "was improvised by civilians who had never handled a hijacked aircraft that attempted to disappear, and by a military unprepared for the transformation of commercial aircraft into weapons of mass destruction"(31). Three major categories of mistaken practice precipitated the tactical failures of that day—each with important practical bearings on the approach to coercion in mass casualty medicine.

First, defense efforts were predicated on several false assumptions. Virtually everyone assumed that hijackers would want to negotiate and seek concessions rather than convert airplanes into weapons. Despite the frequency of suicide attacks in the Middle East, no one in authority seriously considered the possibility of this species of suicide attack occurring in the United States. As a result, planners assumed that any air attack on the United States would come from overseas and that they would have ample time to mount an air defense—an assumption that led to several highly maladaptive protocols. More generally, officials, rescuers, and leaders at all levels were conditioned to believe—despite mountains of contrary evidence—that minimally trained or untrained individuals would panic in emergencies of this magnitude. This assumption precluded them from optimally using important frontline personnel.

Luckily, the terrorists on United 93 also seem to have suffered the illusion that passengers would be immobilized by fear. Several passengers commented to loved ones that terrorists knew they were conversing on cell phones and with each other but didn't care. On other flights, even flight attendants managed to converse on cell phones. American Airlines Flight 11 was the first plane hijacked and the first to crash (into the North Tower of the World Trade Center). Regarding this flight, the 9/11 Commission reports:

> About five minutes after the hijacking began, Betty Ong contacted the American Airlines Southeastern Reservations Office in Cary, North Carolina, via an AT&T airphone to report an emergency aboard the flight. This was the first of several occasions on 9/11 when flight attendants took action outside the scope of their training, which emphasized that in hijacking, they were to communicate with the cockpit crew. The emergency call lasted approximately 25 minutes, as Ong calmly and professionally relayed information about events taking place aboard the airplane to authorities on the ground. (5)

Two flight attendants and a passenger had been stabbed, and they had been told there was a bomb in the cockpit, but Ong and her colleague, flight attendant Amy Sweeney, made multiple calls passing on crucial information—all the time as calm as if they were folding towels. Perhaps unfortunately, the passengers on American 11 remained largely out of the loop—believing that the stabbed individuals were suffering routine medical emergencies. Who knows what resources they could have brought to the situation had they been accurately informed.[2]

The second and third categories of mistaken practice—maladaptive protocols that centralize decisional authority and inefficient information exchange—functioned in negative synergy to vitiate air defense efforts. Officials who were in a position to initiate timely countermeasures often showed excessive concern for establishing or deferring to a chain of command. While they waited for word from above, they delayed communications with other crucial parties, losing precious opportunities for timely intervention. These sorts of mistakes affected the response to each of the four hijackings on September 11. There were also, however, instances where operatives took the initiative to improvise timely actions and communications—outside protocol and the chain of command—and these instances begot the day's most worthwhile official actions. Let us examine some of the details.

The Federal Aviation Administration (FAA) and the North American Aerospace Defense Command (NORAD) are tasked with protecting commercial travelers in America's airspace. Chain of command in the FAA ascends from local air traffic controllers to controllers and managers in regional Traffic *Control* Centers, and from these to the national Air Traffic Control System *Command* Center in Herndon, Virginia. The Command Center reports to the *Operations* Center at FAA headquarters.

NORAD is broken down into sectors, and each of the hijackings on 9/11 occurred in the Northeast Air Defense Sector (NEADS). There are seven NORAD alert sites in the United States, each with two fighters on alert. Two of these alert sites, at Otis Air National Guard Base and Langley Air Force Base, are within NEADS. The protocol for obtaining military assistance in an airline emergency is explained in the 9/11 Commission Report: "If a hijack was confirmed, procedures called for the [FAA] hijack coordinator on duty to contact the Pentagon's National Military Command Center (NMCC) and to ask for a military escort aircraft to follow the flight, report anything unusual, and aid search and rescue in the event of an emergency. The NMCC would then seek approval from the Office of the Secretary of Defense to provide military assistance. If approval was given, the orders would be transmitted down NORAD's chain of command" (17–18). As the 9/11 commissioners report (citing crucial mistaken factual assumptions on which the procedures were based), this protocol was "unsuited in every respect for what was about to happen."

The protocol outlined above did not succeed in producing military notification, much less action, in any of the 9/11 hijackings. Interestingly, the military received timely notice only on the first of the four flights (American 11)—this notification occurring 13 minutes after the plane was known to be hijacked, when a worker at Boston Traffic Control Center broke the chain of command and called NEADS directly, asking them to scramble some fighters. NEADS immediately placed fighters at battle station, but 9 more minutes were lost as the scramble request was processed through the NORAD chain of command. As the fighters took off from Otis Air National Guard Base at 8:46 a.m., American 11 crashed into the North Tower of the World Trade Center (20).

Seven minutes later, a controller at New York Traffic Control Center following United 175 declared, "We may have a hijack." The controller in charge promptly notified a Center manager that she believed United 175 had also been hijacked. The Center manager then tried to notify regional managers, but they were in a meeting and refused to be disturbed. This meeting evidently was focused on the management of American 11—the regional managers being unaware that it had crashed 10 minutes earlier. A few minutes later, between 9:01 and 9:02 a.m., a New York Center manager bypassed the chain of command and called the Herndon Command Center directly—but too late. The scrambled Otis fighters were hovering near New York, but never got the word about United 175, which crashed into the South Tower of the World Trade Center at 9:03 a.m. (21–22).

At about the same time, air traffic controllers at Indianapolis Center were trying to locate American Flight 77. Unlike the CNN-watching public, they were unaware of the other two hijackings, and they assumed that American 77 was suffering from electrical problems. Finally concluding that the plane had crashed, at 9:08 Indianapolis Center asked Langley Search and Rescue to help them look for a downed plane. It was 9:20 a.m. before Indianapolis Center learned of the other two hijackings, and 9:24 a.m. before FAA headquarters learned that American 77 was missing. Because information didn't circulate about the other flights, and controllers consequently assumed that American 77 had crashed, no one until then considered that the plane might be hijacked. Thus the plane, scheduled originally to travel to Los Angeles, traveled undetected for 36 minutes on a course toward Washington, D.C.

As they put together the pieces of this puzzle, a manager at the Herndon Control Center asked FAA headquarters if they wanted a "nationwide ground stop." Executives at headquarters said they needed to discuss the matter first, but Herndon Command Center went ahead and ordered it while they talked. No one at FAA headquarters ever asked for military assistance, though NEADS personnel learned by chance that American 77 was missing when they phoned Washington Center for information about American 11. Langley fighters were deployed, but communications glitches caused them to travel east over the ocean. They were 150 miles away when American 77 crashed into the Pentagon at 9:37 a.m. (24–27).

The fourth hijacking was United Airlines Flight 93—the one that crashed at 10:03 a.m. as passengers charged the cockpit. Cleveland Traffic Control Center tracked the hijacked plane, and as early as 9:36 a.m. asked Herndon Command Center if someone had contacted the military to request fighters. Cleveland Center also said that it was ready to contact a nearby military base to make the request. They were told by the Command Center "that FAA personnel well above them in the chain of command had to make the decision to seek military assistance and were working on the issue." Actually, it was not until 13 minutes later that the topic was even broached at the Command Center, and no one from FAA headquarters contacted the military to pass on information or to request assistance (28–30).

In Washington, D.C., Vice President Cheney never received word of the first flight that crashed in that city, but between 10:10 and 10:15, he received word that another apparently hijacked flight (United 93) was headed there (although in actuality it had crashed by then). When queried, the vice president made the decision to shoot down the incoming aircraft "in about the time it takes a batter to decide to swing." However, as shootdown orders were transmitted through the chain of command, their content changed. By the time orders reached the pilots, they consisted only of authorization to identify and tail the inbound aircraft (41–43).

THE CONTEXT OF TACTICAL DECISIONS ABOUT COERCION IN MASS CASUALTY MEDICINE

Much of this book's focus to this point has been on public deliberation and the dynamics of group decision making in public policy. But as we coalesce the learning points from 9/11, it becomes obvious that tactical leadership is not always about conducting a good discussion. Tactical decisions typically occur under logistic or time constraints that preclude extensive or systematic deliberation. Large-scale public dialogue will usually be unworkable, and occasionally even a hastily conceived council will be too time-consuming to be useful.

Though important medical decisions in the majority of mass casualty events (e.g., epidemics, bombings, hurricanes) are very different from a time-constraint point of view than the aerospace defense decisions on 9/11,[3] some MCM events (especially attacks with $D_1L_1T_2$ agents) are analogous. Even when the window of opportunity is considerably larger, it rarely allows for extensive deliberation or the usual bureaucratic checks and balances. That is why strategists typically make bad tacticians—it is hard for them to lay the protocols aside, especially when adherence to protocol provides the best possible defense against Monday-morning quarterbacks. Thus, in its response to Hurricane Katrina, FEMA proved less efficient than private corporations such as Wal-Mart and Home Depot. While FEMA answered to the Department of Homeland Security—busy with various turf battles and a federal lawsuit in which public workers sought the reversal of rules that would allow the DHS to quickly relocate them in response to strategic and tactical contingencies—Home Depot operated in what journalist Daniel Henninger has called "an alternative universe": "Home Depot's managers answer to flexible procedures; bureaucracies have rules that carry the force of law. In 2004, federal agencies issued 4,100 final rules. . . . Those rules accrete into layers of dos and don'ts, subject to understandably random interpretation by agency rule—keepers of what they might mean. Eventually, no one has an incentive to reform or "shake up" these systems."[4]

The most important similarity between 9/11 aerospace defense and the management of typical MCM events is the occurrence, in both cases, of tactical problems related to unique, unanticipated threats (e.g., suicide hijackings, mutant bacteria, tornado-floods) and the consequent necessity for emergent forms of collective action (in the 9/11 case, direct, expeditious communication and coordination between air traffic controllers and military pilots). The response to these tactical problems requires a nimble, adaptive approach in both national defense and MCM—as we shall observe in considering another illustrative case: terrorist attacks with nerve agents.

When terrorists from the Aum Shinrikyo cult released sarin vapor into a Tokyo subway in 1995, responders were almost wholly unprepared. Though Aum Shinrikyo had deployed the same nerve agent in a courtyard in Matsumoto six months previously (killing seven), officials and medical personnel in Tokyo had not established decontamination protocols or other needed response measures for similar attacks in their jurisdiction. The sarin delivery system employed by the cult was crude, and the concentration it produced was fairly dilute. Hence, all but one of the twelve fatally afflicted commuters was able to get off the train before they died, and some of these died only because they remained on the train after symptoms developed—apparently not wanting to be late for work. Only three mortally injured victims made it to a hospital alive, one dying in an emergency department and the others dying much later from secondary complications. Nevertheless, despite the limited magnitude of the attack, emergency services and hospital emergency departments in Tokyo were overwhelmed.[5]

Within a few hours of the attack, nearby Tokyo hospitals received over 3,500 patients. Due to the failure to decontaminate patients at the scene or on the hospital grounds, many facilities were contaminated, and many emergency workers, physicians, and nurses became ill.[6] Fortunately, the small number of serious casualties produced minimal demand for pharmacological treatments, and supplies of atropine and oximes were adequate.[7]

As with the response to airline hijackings on 9/11, the Tokyo event proceeded very rapidly as officials tasked with protecting public safety floundered or were oblivious. And—again in analogy to 9/11 aerospace defense—the response to chemical casualties in Tokyo was vitiated by false assumptions, maladaptive protocols, and poor information exchange. For example, Tokyo authorities seem to have assumed that, in the event of a hazardous materials accident, it would be possible to contain victims in a warm zone and decontaminate them there. This assumption works for typical industrial accidents, but terrorist attacks with chemical vapors are a wholly different affair. In part because of this false assumption, hospitals created medical protocols that focused on treating casualties, with no defensive contingency for expeditiously decontaminating them before entry into the emergency department. Furthermore, lessons learned in Matsumoto were not imparted to Tokyo officials, and accurate news from the subway didn't reach hospitals until after they were inundated with contaminated casualties.[8]

Distressingly, many similar or identical false assumptions, maladaptive protocols, and inadequate communications plague the U.S. disaster response system today— and many of these liabilities have important consequences for the use of coercion in instances such as a nerve agent attack. When things aren't running smoothly, coercion is frequently seen as the necessary ingredient for reestablishing order.

One common false assumption is that the National Pharmaceutical Stockpile (NPS), which stockpiles atropine and oximes, among other agents that might be used in various disasters, will be helpful in chemical attacks. But things happen too quickly for that to be the case. As exercises such as TopOff have shown, even in slowly developing mass casualty events such as biological attacks, speed of access to the NPS is problematic. More important, perhaps, than the 24-hour delay in getting needed drugs from the NPS to the disaster site are the further delays that occur as the drugs are processed locally (and officials debate how and to whom they should be distributed). In a chemical attack, the window of opportunity would be closed before federal authorities even considered that their help was needed. Adequate stockpiles of nerve agent remedies need to be immediately available to those responding in the field and to physicians and nurses in hospitals and secondary assessment centers. Such provisions are a local affair.

A second false assumption is that all or most of the medical treatment for chemical and biological casualties can be undertaken in hospitals, so long as these hospitals have made adequate provisions for increased "surge capacity" and for sharing their resources in a disaster. But even in relatively puny affairs like the Tokyo sarin attack, this approach is entirely unworkable. Emergency departments in this country routinely operate beyond capacity, feeling besieged as they see 50–200 patients a day.[9] They cannot be tweaked, even with the most concerted preplanning, site expansion, and reinforcement from other hospital personnel, to process thousands of contaminated casualties per hour. Most victims of a nerve gas attack or a biological attack can and should be treated outside the hospital (though treatment at the event site typically will not be possible).

Third, planners and tactical personnel often falsely assume that terrorist attacks will be strongly analogous to non-MCM medical emergencies. Respecting chemical terrorism, this assumption manifests not only in the aforementioned belief that victims should be sent to hospitals, but also in mistaken advice that chemical victims should be treated in accordance with Hazmat[10] protocols. But terrorist attacks with chemical agents are very different than ordinary Hazmat events in that terrorist attacks nearly always will employ vapors or gases (versus liquids with typical Hazmat events), they typically generate far more casualties, and the psychological effects (especially for the rescuers) are usually more severe.

In attacks with $D_1L_1T_2$ agents, such as nerve agents, these false assumptions can lead to unnecessary coercion through several mechanisms. Most disaster plans dictate that rescuers responding to reports of a chemical attack should define a "hot zone" perimeter (the hot zone is an area considered to be dangerously contaminated) and establish a "warm zone" where victims can be decontaminated and a "cold zone" where properly decontaminated patients can receive further medical care or transportation to another facility. As indicated previously in the discussion of mustard agents, full decontamination involves totally undressing and thorough water flushing (e.g., showering). Law enforcement personnel (or perhaps their surrogates) are frequently ordered to prevent yet-to-be-decontaminated victims from leaving the warm zone—by force if necessary.

But this form of coercion is often unnecessary. Asymptomatic contaminated patients who leave the scene of a nerve agent attack do not pose a threat to other persons unless they congregate in an enclosed area (such as an emergency department waiting room). By all means, these victims should be required to decontaminate thoroughly before entering an ambulance or a hospital. But such requirements are not coercive. They are conditions for receiving treatment or entering protected property, and they can be accomplished without imprisoning victims within warm zone boundaries. Furthermore, more than 80 percent of ambulatory casualties can be expected to leave the scene before authorities establish a perimeter (as they did in Tokyo, Nairobi, and other scenes of terrorism). Hence, hospitals and other receiv-

ing facilities will have to protect their boundaries regardless of containment measures attempted by attack-scene authorities.

As with mustard agent attacks, the rationale for forcing nerve agent victims to
remain in the warm zone is prevention of self-harm. Based on the earlier discussion
of PSH in this book, this rationale would justify coercive restraint of nerve agent victims only when there is reason to believe that they cannot make an informed decision on their own *and* that they will suffer significant harm as a result. Both of these
criteria were satisfied in the mustard gas example; neither is likely to apply in typical nerve agent attacks. With nerve agents, seriously contaminated victims will usually show symptoms early and will probably witness other persons collapsing precip-
itously. These factors make it far less likely that they will ignore or disbelieve
announcements about a suspected chemical attack. And, in distinction to the case
with mustard agents, those well enough to leave the scene on their own generally
will not suffer serious harm. Thus, coercion to contain a warm zone is unjustified
in nerve agent vapor attacks. It occurs not only because of a too-robust willingness
to appeal to PSH but also because of the false assumption that these attacks are like
typical, liquid-agent Hazmat events (or mustard agent attacks), where failure to
decontaminate at the scene produces serious harm.

At stake is the mistaken notion that adequate treatment for mass casualty victims
equates with the ordinary standard of care. Logistic barriers and, less frequently, resource shortages, make that impossible in many cases. In most MCM events, the
majority of patients will be minimally afflicted. For instance, in a typical nerve agent
attack, ambulatory victims (e.g., most of the 3,500 patients who streamed into Tokyo
hospitals) require no treatment beyond dry decontamination (i.e., disrobing) and
cogent, understandable discharge instructions. True enough, optimal decontamination includes disrobing and water flushing. However, ambulatory nerve agent vapor
victims decontaminated with disrobing alone virtually always do well. Subsequently,
they can be flushed en masse in a ladder-pipe decontamination system (which can
be constructed with fire trucks), told to visit a secondary assessment center (SAC) for
further evaluation and debriefing, or in some circumstances even told to go home
and shower.[11] Though this approach does not provide the theoretically best medical
care, in large-scale nerve agent attacks these measures would adequately prevent
serious complications and are the only logistically feasible alternatives. From an
MCM perspective, they constitute adequate treatment. And from the perspective of
MCM ethics, they are preferable to coercion—just because they favor public service over logistic simplicity and vindicate public trust by preserving the liberty to
choose between feasible medical options.

Most MCM events are, from the standpoint of time compression, unlike the nerve agent attacks I have used as my primary example. If we are to wield the remedies to nerve agent poisoning effectively, we must get them to patients very quickly, preferably at the scene. In biological terrorism, bombings, natural disasters, and other more typical MCM events, however, immediate treatment is less often a primary objective. Lifesaving field maneuvers such as emergency cricothyrotomy are sometimes an exception, but in many instances these procedures are foregone because they prevent rescuers from executing their primary responsibility—facilitating the flow of salvageable patients toward destinations where they can receive definitive treatment. The greatest challenge in most MCM scenarios arises not so much from time constraints (though these always pertain), or even from personnel or resource shortages (which frequently do not pertain). The challenge arises from getting the right people, properly equipped, to the right places in a fairly expeditious manner and then keeping them mutually apprised so that they can coordinate their efforts.[12]

Personnel shortages are also not the rule. In distinction to MCM exercises, where gathering participants is a challenge, real disasters generate legions of qualified and unqualified volunteers. Finding a way to process and effectively use an excess of such willing participants generally constitutes the primary personnel problem. Nevertheless, once again we see that MCM strategy and tactics are often based on falsely assuming just the opposite. Policy makers who assume that there will be clinician shortages emphasize the necessity of effecting health powers legislation that will enable them to conscript physicians coercively.[13] On the same assumption, some tacticians recommend preventing excess patient/provider ratios by not educating the public in advance about the location of antibiotic distribution centers. In at least one case, experience in MCM exercises was cited as authority for this view.[14]

To deal with the logistical challenges that characterize the tactical management of MCM events, planners in the United States have widely adopted an organizational device known as the Incident Command System (ICS).[15] I now turn to the uses, merits, and possible pitfalls of this device.

TACTICAL DECISIONAL AUTHORITY AND THE INCIDENT COMMAND SYSTEM

The Incident Command System was initially developed by FIRESCOPE[16] in the 1970s to handle large brush and forest fires that require a multijurisdictional response. Based largely on concepts borrowed from the military,[17] the FIRESCOPE version of ICS employs specific mechanisms (command structure, division of labor, staging and sectoring procedures) for handling tactical intra- and inter-organizational coordination, communication, task allocation, and decision making.[18] There are five major areas in the ICS structure: Command, Operations, Logistics, Planning, and Finance. Each area has an individual officer in charge. In the Command Post, the Incident Commander is assisted by Safety, Liaison, and Information officers. Overall command, and command in the specific areas, is transmitted through a "bump up and down" protocol. For instance, the highest ranking officer who is first on the scene becomes the initial incident commander. As higher ranking officers arrive and decide their services are needed (or not needed), the command may (or may not) "bump up" to them, then perhaps "bump down" again when they leave. The various areas are mobilized in a step-wise fashion as they are needed. Hence, not every area is mobilized in every disaster.

Since its inception, the ICS has undergone numerous modifications, both within fire-fighting organizations and as non-fire-fighting organizations tailor it for their specific purposes. For more than two decades, it has been the most prominent organizational framework for community disaster response—though often the communities and organizations that claim to use it know little more about ICS than that it requires them to designate "someone in charge."[19] Because of these modifications, adaptations, and misunderstandings, one can no longer assume any particular or precise denotation to mentions of an "Incident Command System."

In the response to major disasters, including mass casualty events, individual organizations may employ their own internal incident command structure (e.g., hospitals may have intraorganizational response plans based on HEICS, the "Hospital Emergency Incident Command System") while also serving in various units (medical responders come under "Operations") and sectors of a more general incident command. Because ICS is a tactical system, the scene Incident Commander generally will be in communication with officials from a larger strategic body, such as an Emergency Operations Center (EOC). Unfortunately, the typical ICS contains relatively little guidance for communication and integration with such strategic organizations.

Despite the presence of a significant body of research casting doubt on the effectiveness of ICS for disasters other than forest and brush fires,[20] and despite a total absence of systematic research that compares ICS to other possible organizational frameworks,[21] the 9/11 Commission states that ICS is a "proven framework" for responding to forensic and public health emergencies—strongly recommending that it be used in all jurisdictions and that its adoption become a criterion for federal funding.[22] By "proven," they can only mean that it has been widely used, and in some circumstances at least, it seems to have worked pretty well. With respect to this modest standard of proof, they are certainly right. In any case, it seems that—given critical assessment and much-needed revision—the ICS is a potentially effective organizational framework that, whether we like it or not, is here to stay.

One of the supposed virtues of ICS is that everyone knows—or theoretically should know—where the highest tactical decisional authority lies. It lies with the Incident Commander, a position ultimately filled in most full-fledged disasters by the senior fire department or police department official. This clarity can be an asset so long as rescuers understand that the "highest decisional authority" does not imply "the only decisional authority" or "the authority who needs to sign off on all significant decisions." Even though the chain of command is arguably more efficient in ICS than in joint FAA/NORAD aerospace defense, it is often elaborate enough that it would be disastrous to assume that all important decisions need to be cycled through the ICS chain of command.[23]

Because that is precisely what has happened on numerous occasions, and precisely what some ICS advocates seem to be recommending, the model has come under fire from disaster researchers.[24] Quarantelli remarks that a "strong tendency among disaster managers is to think that because they have not planned for or are not in control of something, it cannot be good."[25] The contention is that an underlying "command and control" philosophy in ICS begets just the sort of maladaptive delays, equivocation, information loss, and poor information sharing that we observed when command-and-control habits manifested themselves in the 9/11 hijackings. As an alternative to the command-and-control model, Quarantelli recommends what he has variously called an "emergent resource model," or a "coordinative and resource management model,"[26] that emphasizes coordination rather than control. Though ICS proponents all agree that "coordination" is critically important, they frequently use the term in a way that diverges from Quarantelli's.

Quarantelli identifies three views of coordination. According to the first, coordination occurs when groups inform one another of what they are doing. This is not genuine coordination because there is no judgment about how the various groups can complement one another in service of their mutual end: protecting persons and property in a manner that is as efficient and unobtrusive as possible. The second view equates coordination with centralized organization and decision making—a view Quarantelli attributes to many disaster planners. But central direction does not guarantee smooth interaction—and often, as we have seen, it thwarts it. The third view, endorsed by Quarantelli, is that coordination consists of "mutually agreed upon cooperation about how to carry out particular tasks."[27] These mutual agreements for cooperation will not always be made in advance (though advance arrangements are sometimes immensely helpful). To the contrary, they often occur on an ad hoc basis as circumstances dictate—and they are often made at low or intermediate levels of decisional authority. For instance, most of the search and rescue in actual disasters is undertaken by civilian bystanders and volunteers who get to the scene first.[28]

In describing his emergent resource model, Quarantelli refers to an example that is particularly relevant for mass casualty medicine:

> In disasters when there are a fair number of casualties coming into hospitals, the institutions slowly get overwhelmed by the number of cases in their emergency rooms. Now in terms of organizational structure, overall decisions about patient intake, the clearing of beds, and other functions are to be done by the administrative staff. Thus, information first goes up to the top of the bureaucracy and then orders proceed down through the chain of command. However, in disasters what often happens is a decentralization of decision making. Thus, the Chief Nurse at the Emergency Room of one hospital—seeing it being slowly overwhelmed by incoming victims—will place a phone call to a Chief Nurse in another hospital, and ask the other nurse about their load. If the other hospital can take the overload, the first nurse will redirect subsequent patients to the second hospital, something which even if it is in the hospital planning usually is the responsibility of the chief administrator. Actually this decentralization in decision making is very functional. Of course to this day there are some administrators who do not know why their hospital stopped getting victims and why they were able to handle the patient load that they had. The crucial decision was made at a much lower level than usual in the organization.[29]

In an age of EMTALA, it is perhaps less likely that nurses would take the initiative in such ways.[30] But Quarantelli's point is a good one. Effective MCM requires malleable organizational structures and protocols, sometimes fashioned by individuals who are closely proximate to the circumstances and tactical challenges that make rapid changes necessary.

This sort of openness to innovation and improvisation is not incompatible with ICS. But it requires that leaders mold their notions of "command" around a robust concept of "coordination" rather than reducing coordination to a mere manifestation of central control. In Quarantelli's example of nurses coordinating patient flow, it would be helpful if news of these adjustments got quickly to EMS and other units involved in the disposition of casualties. One of the functions of the command center is to ensure that such communications are undertaken quickly and efficiently. Another function of an incident command center should be to monitor the flow of events resulting from lower-level decisions and intervene when some of these decisions are clearly incongruent or otherwise maladaptive. It would be little trouble, and possibly salient, if the chief nurse sent news of her decision through the hospital information system, where it could then be accessed by the hospital commander. In some instances, the commander would have information bearing on this decision that the nurse lacked, and on the basis of this information might choose to modify or reverse the nurse's arrangements or to tweak the system in other areas so that things coordinate a little better. Viewed in this manner, the command center maintains useful elements of command and control while focusing on its more central task: coordination.

The transportation protocol mutually enacted by the nurses in the example above is an illustration of emergent social action that enhances coordination. By "emergent social action" I denote activities manifesting novel forms of social organization, begot by novel circumstances, and modifying those circumstances for better or worse. Some emergent action is undertaken by individuals who are members of preexisting organizations designated to participate in the disaster response — this activity typically occurring as these organizations extend their operations,[31] and some emergent action is undertaken by civilian bystanders and others who have no particularly relevant organizational affiliations. Sometimes emergent action — by designated participants or otherwise — is adaptive. Sometimes it is not.

Any disaster plan, and any interpretation of the Incident Command System, that fails to take account of emergent social action and the unique forms of cooperation it entails, will at best be largely irrelevant (since emergent behavior is ubiquitous) — and at worst be lethal. Even military leaders understand that command-and-control structures frequently (and by necessity) give way to innovation and improvisation in combat: "No plan survives contact with the enemy." The best military leaders always emphasize improvisational skills in training. And so should disaster response planners, who, unlike military campaigners, can look forward to dealing with legions of outside organizations, bystanders, volunteers, and others who insistently offer their helping hands.

These "helping hands" will be active whether they are wanted or not. Creativity and tact in facilitating their involvement augments MCM efforts in several ways — not the least of which being that it enhances public solidarity and trust, which, as previously noted, are crucial elements in cultivating public cooperation. And public cooperation is the ultimate prophylaxis against coercion.

TACTICAL LEADERSHIP AND COERCION

Good tactical decisions about coercion are decisions that effectively integrate potentially applicable values — especially security and liberty. Ideally, conflicts between these values can be prevented or mitigated so that they are more aligned than at odds. When, however, they remain irretrievably at odds, tactical leaders must strive toward a decent balance. In either case, effective tactical leadership requires a well-developed capacity of practical judgment.

Practical judgment is the virtue of integrating numerous related and sometimes countervailing considerations into a plan of action that satisfies needs, norms, and other values in a good way. Instead of saying "in a good way," I might have used loftier language, like "in the best possible way," or "in a manner that maximally enhances the likelihood of overall success." But practical judgment is a practical concept. One of its characteristics is its qualitative—almost aesthetic—nature. It brings together apples, oranges—and, if need be, fried chicken livers—to produce a concoction that seems relatively palatable, given the circumstances. Just as there is no "best possible way" to create an entree, there is no "best possible way" to make any particular tactical decision.

For tactical decisions in mass casualty medicine—especially decisions about the use of coercion—recipes give way to less precise guidelines. This book has already produced some very general guidelines about tactical decision making. Legitimacy in this domain, we earlier concluded, is a function of good reasons (GRL). That is, good tactical judgments will be based on good reasons, mixing an understanding of general and particular facts with appeals to ethical norms, laws, practices, and precedents. We also observed that what counts as good reasons will vary in different jurisdictions, just as geography, customs, laws, and practices will vary from place to place. Good reasons legitimacy about value judgments, we thus concluded, is optimally predicated to some degree on the prior deliberation of the local public.

With respect to good judgment in tactical decisions about coercion, this means that decision makers will to some degree have internalized the values that emerge in public deliberation. Of course, the public's ability to accurately anticipate a future disaster and to deliberate at length about its management is sharply limited. Only general guidelines will be available. This entails, as we have observed, that tactical decision making needs to be highly adaptive—to nuance and to the rapidly changing, novel circumstances that make mass casualty medicine such a monumental challenge. Perhaps we can flesh out these ideas a bit by considering specific qualities of a good tactical leader.

First, the tactical leader needs to understand and interpret publicly issued guidelines in a manner that reflects the original spirit and intentions of those who framed them. In the first chapter scenario, where Marcia Welby stretched and contorted the public health law to justify quarantining her tularemia patient, this type of understanding was not in evidence. In essence, she allowed particular personal and professional values to trump what should have been a more fundamental commitment to public service—a commitment that requires, among other things, the will to up-hold public decisions and guidelines insofar as these are discernable and arise from legitimate sources.[32]

A second necessary quality for tactical managers is that they be well-informed fac-tually. There is no excuse for holding to stagnant, thoroughly repudiated dogmas (such as: "ordinary citizens typically panic and are uncooperative in a disaster"; "de-contamination of gas or vapor chemical weapons victims is the same as decontami-nation of liquid chemical exposures"; "it is usually possible to perform onsite triage operations for the majority of disaster victims"; or "search and rescue operations and transportation of casualties are generally done by trained rescuers and EMS").[33] Belief in such falsehoods may well be more prevalent than overly pronounced con-cern for security as a cause of unnecessary coercion in MCM.

Third, the tactical leader needs to be well rehearsed in tactical decision making. One point that is emphasized repeatedly by disaster researchers is that tactical train-ing should focus on problem solving, coordinating decisions, and accomplishing tasks, rather than on establishing a particular organizational structure. Experience can help,[34] but individuals who have worked more than a handful of mass casualty situations are few in number. Training and simulations are usually the only focused training alternatives. These should be executed without advance notice and should not proceed by scripted scenarios. But such advice is infrequently heeded, as Quar-antelli observes:

> Disaster planners sometimes undertake a disaster exercise or simulation of some kind. But the planners will write out a very elaborate script for how the actors and organiza-tions should perform in the exercise or drill. Unfortunately, this is the wrong way to pro-ceed. Pat or packaged solution for potential problems or difficulties should not be pro-vided. Instead, those in a disaster exercise should be made to think about the questions or issues they will be faced with in actual disasters, . . . especially the tactical matters they will have to consider. In other words, disaster simulations or tests should teach offi-cials the questions rather than the answers, provide more of a roadmap than a script or blueprint.[35]

Recently, the federal government spent millions of dollars on the scripted TopOff exercises (the third TopOff being executed at about the time of this writing). Before TopOff2, the *Wall Street Journal* published a "Calendar of the Crisis" that included comprehensive details about when the attacks would occur, which agents would be used, how many casualties would be produced—and even a timetable for a "diver-sionary" dirty bomb (as if realistic training for diversionary strikes could be under-taken where everyone has advance knowledge of the details and purpose of the strike).[36] This sort of exercise has little or no value for cultivating the kind of adaptability that tactical leaders need most.

Fourth, then, the tactical leader needs to be an adaptive thinker. Instead of focusing on bureaucratic questions like "Who is in charge?" or "Which organization is officially responsibility for this task?" the adroit tactical leader thinks contextually. "What needs to be done?" "What resources are needed, and where?" "What is going well and what needs to be done better?" With respect to the use of coercion, tacticians should always be asking: "How is it possible to achieve this objective without the use of force or, at least, with minimal coercion?"

I am aware of no systematic data pertaining to the proclivities of tactical leaders toward coercion during MCM. It is disconcerting, however, to witness the glee some high-ranking officials project over the prospect of using force in a public emergency. I recall a prospective incident commander who announced that, should there be a chemical attack downtown, he would immediately seize control of the nearest hotel so that he could use its showers for decontamination. This tactic—like so many maladaptive decisions that employ coercion—manifests love of power, unadulterated by practical judgment. Seizing a hotel and getting casualties processed through its labyrinth of discontinuous showers would be a logistical nightmare—and especially unnecessary, given that the task could be accomplished quickly, efficiently, and without coercion by employing a ladder-pipe decontamination system (LDS), augmented by a corridor system for casualties on gurneys (and perhaps for those who refuse the LDS on grounds of modesty).[37] The most immediate decontamination objective for ambulatory, asymptomatic victims at the scene of most vapor/gas chemical attacks will be to get them undressed quickly. Once they are undressed, they are generally better than 90 percent decontaminated.[38]

That leads to a fifth characteristic of good tactical leaders. They are publicly responsive. One of the problems that might pertain in efforts to move victims through an LDS is that some (or many) would object to the public nudity that most LDS protocols prescribe. The guidelines call for "disrobing totally"—and that means that even underwear must go. So in cases such as mustard gas attacks (but, again, not nerve gas attacks), where mandatory decontamination may be justified, should victims be forced to remove their underwear or forced to stay at the scene until they are suitably naked? For the publicly responsive tactician, the answer is "of course not." The protocol requiring total disrobing is based, once again, on the questionable notion that vapor and gas attacks should be handled like typical liquid Hazmat events. To press the issue on a matter like this would be foolhardy—provoking distrust, noncooperation, and a flurry of more serious problems that follow from these. In a vapor attack it is almost inconceivable that underwear that was well covered by outerwear would get significantly contaminated.[39] Victims should be advised that the best and safest option is to totally disrobe, including underwear. If some of them insist otherwise, they should be granted the prerogative. Perhaps the most important tactical device in getting reluctant patients to disrobe quickly (time lost in cajoling could be crucial) is to offer them personal decontamination kits, which contain plastic overgarments (large trash bags also suffice), affording privacy while the garments underneath are removed and placed in separate bags.[40] Recently, when I suggested to the leader of a decontamination task force that we make these kits available, he responded that he was (and in a disaster would be) busy with more important considerations and that he hardly had the time, money, or inclination to prepare for actions that indulge victims' modesty. But in the matters of preventing coercion and facilitating patient flow, the kits could play a crucial role. They are cheap, effective, and easy to use. Tactical leaders need to make time for such measures.

Another element of public responsiveness is the willingness to involve citizens in planning and, when the right circumstances arise, in operations. To some degree the former is inevitable, because the public seems to be demanding it.[41] But much more could be done. In TopOff2, for instance, volunteers were recruited only from specific high schools and senior centers (planners cited security reasons).[42] And the news media was not involved at all—planners choosing instead to hire contractors to form a virtual news network.[43] This omission deeply vitiated the relevance and scope of the exercise, since news media are a crucial asset for passing information to citizens and officials alike.[44] Recall that on 9/11, most federal officials learned about the hijackings on CNN, and air traffic controllers who didn't watch CNN often were among the last to get the word.

The news media should be exploited. Yet too often interorganizational barriers to information gathering and maladaptive media habits detract from their contribution. According to researchers at the Disaster Research Center (DRC), important interorganizational problems include denial of access to the impacted area, limited disclosure of relevant information to media reporters, limited access to emergency managers, lack of regularly scheduled press briefings, and difficulties in verifying information. Regarding the internal workings of news media, there is frequently excessive attention to warning, evacuation, short-term sheltering, and impact behavior, with less attention to casualty care; provision of food, clothing, and human services; and the restoration of essential services. Interestingly, there is almost a total lack of coverage of search and rescue activities. The DRC researchers hypothesize that this omission is related to the fact that search and rescue activities are often ad hoc, emergent activities for which information is not available on the usual "beat" sources centering around the command post. They are also concerned that mass media, especially television, often spin their stories in a way that reinforces mistaken popular beliefs. This tendency is related to the penchant for reporting incidents that are dramatic but actually uncommon, thus perpetuating myths about the prominence in disasters of looting, panic, martial law, disaster shock, increasing crime, massive shelter utilization, mass evacuation, and victim helplessness.[45] As observed earlier, this dynamic was in evidence during Hurricane Katrina.

Most mass and local media organizations do not include disaster preparations in their planning and training. Like citizens and local officials, local media tend to have a strong proprietary relationship to their disasters. Many (especially in electronic media) are open to partnering with disaster responders to enhance the flow of crucial information before and during mass casualty events,[46] thus helping to create involved and informed citizens who will be more cooperative, more helpful, and less prone to the sort of irrationality and maladaptive impulses that beget the need for coercion. However, such media-responder partnerships have not been widely cultivated.

Other mass communications sources, besides the news media, can also help MCM managers to elicit adaptive public behavior. Recall the importance on 9/11 of cell phones in allowing citizens and airline crew to pass on information crucial to aerospace defense. They also could have been pivotal in the evacuation of the World Trade Center. However, because telephone operators were not in the informational loop, they were unaware that there could be no rooftop evacuations, and they were not informed when planners decided that the buildings needed to be quickly evacuated. Hence, they frequently dispersed the standard, cookbook advice to callers, telling them to stay put or to make their way to the rooftop. Such advice often proved fatal. In its commentary on these and other tactical evacuation blunders, 9/11 commissioners write: "One clear conclusion of September 11 is that individual civilians need to take responsibility for maximizing the probability that they will survive, should disaster strike."[47] Much of the onus on tactical leaders is to help civilians to help themselves. Likely sources of information for afflicted individuals need to be identified, then exploited by ensuring that the information is timely and correct.

A sixth characteristic, then, of effective tactical leaders is that they will use available personnel and resources in a manner that exploits the adaptive capacities of both civilians and those officially under their command. To some degree this objective necessitates that disaster managers help in the cultivation of adaptive habits *before* disaster strikes. Disaster researchers know that if you want an integrated response during an emergency, the best thing to do is integrate things during the routine.[48] From an interagency perspective, it is important that disaster roles be allocated, when possible, in ways that allow disaster workers to use and adapt the skills they have developed during non-emergencies. Likewise, "role complementarity"—the quality of linking the roles of individuals whose roles are commonly linked in routine situations—should also be cultivated where possible.[49]

From an interagency perspective, establishing congenial, cooperative day-to-day relationships with other organizations is far more important than producing formal disaster-specific cooperative arrangements or operating procedures. Turf wars invariably lead to poor coordination, but such battles are uncommon where relations were good prior to disaster operations.[50] Given a spirit of mutual cooperation and a focus on coordinating activities rather than divvying command, the heterogeneity and variability that public, private, and volunteer organizations bring to a disaster can be a great asset and are perhaps the most reliable way of ensuring that a broad range of local conditions, habits, and circumstances are accounted for in the disaster response.[51]

Quarantelli advises that officials coordinating organizational and community responses could make a good start "by emphasizing co-operation rather than control or insisting that 'someone be in charge.'" He continues: "Much will depend on the tact and sensitivity of key officials, and the willingness to de-emphasize organizational claims of leadership by stressing actions necessary for the greater community good. Appeals to larger symbols and humanitarian concerns can move people and groups to co-operate, especially at the height of a major community disaster."[52]

Ultimately, a good tactical leader is far less apt to resort to coercion than an inept leader, because the superior leader will have made a career out of forging close relationships between parties that are destined for cooperative engagement should disaster arise. Heeding the Aristotelian maxim that one attains a prudent balance between polar extremes by aiming at the more difficult pole, the tactical leader trains both self and others to attend to liberties that are easily forgotten in times of emergency and high emotion. That does not mean that coercion is out of the question. It means that coercion will be avoided wherever possible—and that disaster preparedness efforts will focus intently on innovations that decrease the likelihood that coercion will be needed.

Effective disaster management is more akin to solving a puzzle than it is to enacting a protocol.[53] A crucial part of the puzzle is figuring how to get people to act adaptively on their own—without the threat of force.

CHAPTER SEVEN

Decisions for Particular Coercive Actions

Perhaps the most salient general advice one can give high-level tacticians about coercion in mass casualty medicine is that it can be avoided by delegating some of their decisional authority to frontline personnel—including a degree of latitude even for private-sector experts and untrained civilians. Coercive decisions themselves and their enforcement, however, typically remain within the purview of designated officials and should rarely be delegated outside that pale. The officials who make and enact such decisions should be accountable—not merely in the sense of acting responsibly and in an official capacity, but also in the sense that they should expect punitive measures when they violate the law or exhibit poor judgment.

DECISIONS BY NONMEDICAL PERSONNEL FOR PARTICULAR COERCIVE ACTIONS

Sometimes civilians will attempt to address or forestall a mass casualty event by enacting their own coercive measures, as was the case with the "shotgun quarantines" of the yellow fever era.[1] Such measures are dangerous, almost always wrongheaded, and can be avoided by competent disaster management. They are also uncommon—notwithstanding the widespread myth that social chaos, looting, vigilantism, and other signs of lawlessness frequently erupt during disasters. To the contrary, crime rates, including burglary and theft, typically *decrease* amid disaster. Noting this fact, Auf der Heide writes: "One reason people refuse to evacuate in disasters is to protect their property. It is also ironic that security measures undertaken to 'prevent looting' can prevent residents from salvaging property that is exposed to the elements by the disaster. Finally, overzealous police and security guards manning road-blocks set up to keep looters out sometimes prevent the entry of legitimate disaster-response personnel."[2] If we want to prevent citizens from taking the law into their own hands, we could start by limiting the steady misinformation about looting, violence, and social disorder.

In forensic mass casualty medicine (i.e., medical preparation and response to mass casualty events that result from intentional aggression), community leaders and law enforcement personnel confront somewhat novel and sometimes monumentally difficult problems. It is unwise to add to these increased demands by assigning unnecessary tasks such as policing warm zone boundaries and cordoning off neighborhoods to prevent looting. Above all, public officials should be taught that mass casualty events require the same level of professionalism, good judgment, and accountability as do ordinary situations.

Critics such as Annas are correct, I think, in opposing the clause in the Model State Emergency Health Powers Act that states that public officials will not be held accountable for their actions unless the infringement manifests "gross negligence or willful misconduct." When persons are granted extensive powers to restrain (e.g., mandatory examination and treatment), imprison (e.g., isolation and quarantine), impress (e.g., involuntary conscription of health care workers), and otherwise violate the ordinary civil liberties of innocent citizens, this power should be wielded with caution. Should coercion be enacted cavalierly, punishment is in order. In some circumstances justifiable decisions to enact coercion are best made with the presumption that there will be negative consequences for the decision maker (just as there are negative consequences for the victims of coercion). Such a state of affairs is not unprecedented.

Consider torture, for example. Many national and international organizations and charters have called for an absolute legal prohibition against the use of torture—including cases where national security or many lives are at stake. The justification for this ban is based in part on a causal slippery slope argument. Once we acknowledge the legality of torture, it seems inevitable that the practice will be abused (as allegedly it has been in America's recent war on terror). Yet only the most ardent (and dangerous) deontologist would argue that the decision to torture a person is morally wrong in every conceivable case. If, for instance, we are certain that a person has schemed to kill millions of people (for instance, by placing a 10 kiloton nuclear bomb that will detonate in Manhattan) and justifiably confident that this person will divulge information on how to prevent the detonation if and only if he is tortured, then there is a moral obligation to torture. Opponents of torture rightly argue that such scenarios are fleetingly unlikely—for one thing, because it is not clear that torture is a good or efficient means of extracting accurate information. But in theory at least, there are scenarios in which the refusal to use torture would be morally reprehensible. In such instances, the person who undertakes to torture should expect recriminations—even in the face of the moral rightness of their decision. With so many lives at stake, the willingness of public officials who torture enemies to also serve jail time is expected, as an act of courage and loyalty.

Part of the strong moral appeal of Abraham Lincoln as a national icon is that he displayed just this form of courage during the War between the States. It is ironic that Lincoln—whose deepest political sympathies always remained with an American Whig party founded on its opposition to excessive executive power—expanded executive power to an unprecedented degree in the defense of a moral principle he held to be higher and even more politically fundamental than the division of powers. Throughout the war, Lincoln felt destined to die for his transgression, and he seemed at times to consider this price to be a reasonable and inevitable consequence for his violation of constitutional principles.

Perhaps it would be folly to expect as much from those who make and enact coercive decisions in mass casualty medicine. But some degree of willingness for self-sacrifice, especially in circumstances that require authorities to demand extreme sacrifice from others, is necessary for genuine moral and political authority. Without question, involuntary isolation and quarantine, mandatory medical examination, perhaps even conscription, are necessary in some circumstances (though, again, these measures would rarely if ever be needed if political leaders and public officials enacted prudent disaster response measures). What is not acceptable is that disaster preparations should focus on establishing comfortable mechanisms for enacting these coercive measures without fear of recrimination.[3] Our focus should instead be on ensuring that they rarely happen.

DECISIONS BY MEDICAL PERSONNEL FOR
PARTICULAR COERCIVE ACTIONS

Consider the following scenario:

Denver, Colorado, experiences a sudden outbreak of pneumonic plague. Almost a thousand cases appear in two days, with several precipitous deaths. Epidemiologists quickly discern that Yersinia pestis *was disseminated through the ventilation system at a rock concert three days before the first case. Despite efforts to contact and administer doxycycline and/or streptomycin to everyone present at the concert and their close contacts, plague infection spreads quickly. Within a week there are 10,000 cases and more than 1,000 deaths. Dr. Bill Adams, a Denver internist, is contacted by the governor's office. The governor has declared a state of emergency, and her public health officers have designated Dr. Adams's clinic as a center for evaluating individuals with known or suspected Yersinia exposures. Dr. Adams and several clinician volunteers (members of a Disaster Medical Assistance Team under the National Disaster Medical System) are assigned to work alternating 12-hour shifts. They are to sort each of their ambulatory patients into one of three categories: (1) category one patients are ill, presumably with Yersinia; (2) category two patients are ill but the illness is probably not Yersinia; and (3) category three patients are not ill. Patients in category one will be housed in a building across the street (a converted nursing home) and treated with antibiotics plus additional needed medical treatments. Category two patients will be sent to another facility with medical care as needed. Those in category three will be sent home on antibiotics (with daily visits from public health personnel). The Denver newspaper reports that several patients have been mistakenly triaged to category one and subsequently acquired fatal Yersinia infections, despite antibiotic treatments. Though most patients seem to respond to antibiotics, this development suggests that an antibiotic-resistant strain of Yersinia pestis has emerged.[4]*

Now suppose Dr. Adams evaluates a patient that does not fit neatly into any of the three categories. This particular patient is only slightly ill, with decreased energy and mild pharyngitis. Though these signs could be early manifestations of plague, it is equally likely, given the patient's history, that they are merely symptoms of a mild viral upper respiratory infection (URI), seasonal allergies, or stress. Though this patient might be triaged to category one, a decision that would result in coercive detainment, it is also possible to choose either of the other categories. Category two is justified if Dr. Adams rules that the illness is probably URI. Category three is justified if Dr. Adams rules that the symptoms are insufficiently severe to count as an "illness." Which choice, in this case, is most appropriate?

As with tactical decisions, the quality of this decision for individual action will hinge on Dr. Adams's practical judgment. Recall that practical judgment is the virtue of integrating numerous related and sometimes countervailing considerations into a plan of action that satisfies needs, norms, and other values in a good way. As with other decision makers who must decide about coercion, to judge prudently in this situation Dr. Adams must balance conflicting values of security and liberty. In this case, the conflict between security and liberty might well be viewed as a conflict between the individual interests of his patient (who would be safest if triaged to category three) and the aggregate interests of other persons (who would be safest if the patient were triaged to category one). To cultivate a fully functional capacity for practical judgment, Dr. Adams requires both (1) an ethical rationale to guide particular decisions such as this one, and (2) an ethical ideal that will sustain him through the emotionally tumultuous trials of frontline service in such an unfamiliar, tragic, and bewildering situation. In the remainder of this concluding chapter, we address these requirements.

THE PROBLEM OF BALANCING INDIVIDUAL INTEREST AND AGGREGATE INTEREST

The ethical ideal and more or less firmly entrenched habit in ordinary clinical medicine (OCM) is to attend to the interests of individual patients. This focus on beneficence is regarded by some as medicine's overarching moral principle.[5] However, there are exceptions that suggest that this principle is not supreme. In most states, for instance, physicians must report gunshot or knife wounds and certain sexually transmitted diseases even if the best interests of the patient would be served by keeping these facts confidential. Physicians also may be obligated to refer noncooperative patients with certain infectious diseases to public health authorities for directly observed treatment.[6]

In mass casualty medicine (MCM), there is a transition in emphasis toward the service of particular aggregate interests. As noted in the first chapter, MCM adopts a Rescue Paradigm (RP) that focuses on maximizing aggregate survival while minimizing aggregate morbidity. In view of moral dilemmas such as Dr. Adams's, we might ask if there are exceptions to this principle as well. And such, indeed, seems to be the case. We earlier argued that liberty issues still pertain under RP, and that sometimes crucial liberty issues will prevail over relatively trivial public health considerations.

The existence of exceptions to the rules of patient beneficence in OCM and maximizing aggregate morbidity-limited survival in MCM prove that neither of these rules functions as a fundamental overriding ethical principle in the given contexts. If there is such a fundamental ethical principle, in medicine or elsewhere, this principle will not change as circumstances vary and will not be susceptible to exceptions. Insofar as it is "fundamental," it will dictate changes in the equilibrium between other principles, while itself remaining constant. Furthermore, if there were no more fundamental principle than clinical beneficence or maximizing aggregate morbidity-limited survival, then there could be no basis for justifying a temporary transition from one to the other during a mass casualty event.[7]

What, then, is the fundamental ethical basis for clinical practice? And how, we might ask, is such a principle even possible, given the deeply entrenched moral pluralism that characterizes democratic polities such as the United States? Before I offer an answer to this question, two prevalent but inadequate responses will be considered.

One response derives from the moral philosophy of Immanuel Kant. His fundamental ethical principle is expressed in the "categorical imperative," which he articulates as follows: "I ought never to act except in such a way that I can also will that my maxim become a universal law." For Kant, this principle justifies any particular decision for individual action.[8] In applying the categorical imperative, Dr. Adams would ask: "Am I acting on a maxim that I would accept as a universal law—that is, as a maxim that all other physicians should apply in their treatment of individual patients?" There are numerous maxims that Dr. Adams might consider, and these include (but are not limited to): (1) any patient that has a reasonable chance of having contracted plague should be triaged to category one, or (2) any patient who has a reasonable but not overwhelming chance of having contracted plague, but who would be better off in category two or three, should be triaged to one of these latter categories, depending on the extent to which they are ill. Obviously, the first of these possible maxims is superior as candidate for universal law, since the second maxim defeats the purpose of triage.

Yet there are glaring weaknesses in this approach. First, the categorical imperative is insufficiently responsive to the reality of ethical pluralism. Kant never demonstrates the rightness of his device over and against competing decisional principles grounded in diverging moral visions (for instance, those that reject Kant's assumption that ethical rightness must be an expression of pure practical reason). Thus, not only is his fundamental principle deeply susceptible to criticism, but he also lacks a universal ethical basis for determining the manner in which the categorical imperative will balance competing values. Second, the method of formulating maxims as candidates for universal law does not leave much room for the consideration of context. But practical reason, most would argue, is highly context-sensitive. Dr. Adams must probe deeply into specific matters such as his patient's degree of illness, proclivity to abide by clinical instructions after discharge, extant social determinants of health, and the relative emphasis on security versus liberty in the given jurisdiction.

A second response reflects the philosophy of utilitarianism. Here the fundamental ethical principle for individual action is maximization of the overall good, conceived as the aggregate of individual goods, or as the application of a rule that, when adhered to strictly, will maximize the aggregate good. Because the utilitarian typically recognizes that the comprehensive good for humans consists in more than mere morbidity-limited survival, many utilitarians would acknowledge some leeway for Dr. Adams in acting on behalf of individual patients, even when aggregate morbidity-limited survival is not likely to be maximized. John Stuart Mill, for instance, was a utilitarian who thought that individual freedom was a crucial determinant of individual good. He might condone triage to category three because of its liberty-preserving consequences.

The utilitarian principle, like the categorical imperative, is insufficient in the face of ethical pluralism. It requires agreement on an operative concept of the individual good. But as we have seen, that is just the sort of thing that ethical pluralism precludes. Liberty, for instance, seems to be a crucial determinant of the good life for some individuals but not for others. Concepts like "happiness" and "maximal fulfillment of individual interests" are more promising than wealth or health parameters as markers of the individual good, just because they are ambiguous enough to accommodate a large plurality of diverging particular moral visions. But the ambiguity of these concepts precludes their usefulness in a calculus aimed at estimating the relative value of likely outcomes. And the inability to effectively compare likely outcomes greatly impairs the utility of the utilitarian principle.

Both Kantianism and utilitarianism suffer from ethical shortsightedness. Kantianism focuses on rules or maxims to the exclusion of considerations about outcomes, while utilitarianism focuses on outcomes without much thought about the intrinsic importance of rules and maxims. The result for Kantianism is that it is in practice too legalistic. Kant, for instance, would forbid lying, even when a lie could save countless innocents from torture and death at the hands of an evil malefactor. For utilitarianism, the dysfunction manifests from a too hard-and-fast division between ends (which are regarded as outcomes to be maximized) and means (which are important only insofar as they are connected to outcomes). Because utilitarianism divorces means from ends, it is frequently described as a species of "consequentialism"—"ends" being equated with "consequences." But equal consequences do not always signify ethically equivalent actions. Most persons regard it as better, for instance, to achieve good outcomes through truthfulness than through lying—even if the final result is the same.

There is a superior approach to balancing individual versus aggregate interests, which will be briefly developed in the next section. This approach, like utilitarianism, is oriented toward an end. However, unlike utilitarianism, it does not strictly divorce ends from means. The end, on this view, is ethical reality integrated—not some feature of reality captured through abstraction and a snapshot in time. It includes both "outcomes" and the rules, procedures, attitudes, desires, talents, and habits that operate in their production (thus, it is not accurately described as a species of consequentialism). This approach dates back to Aristotle and beyond, and ethicists call it "teleology."[9]

CIVIC TELEOLOGY

Any complete and comprehensive moral teleology is deeply imbedded in a worldview—replete with particular metaphysical, ethical, and cultural commitments. Because it aspires to the radical tolerance of indifference (described in chapter 3), the pluralistic democratic polis cannot legitimately canonize such a full-fledged moral teleology. In an earlier essay I argued for "an austere Lamarckian framework" for a practical teleology—one far less robust in content than a complete and comprehensive teleology.[10] I now believe this framework also contains too much content to adequately circumscribe a civic teleology within a polity committed to the ideal of radical tolerance. It may be a compelling personal ideal and adaptable to many diverse moral communities, but it is not universally adaptable, and it requires more than basic civic morality can sanction.

All of this is not to imply that the pluralistic polis has no ends or that its ends are somehow content-free. Recall that the radically indifferent state is not a neutral state. To construct a useful but sufficiently austere civic teleology, one must identify the common values that bind members of a polity. These include: (1) common values that cause civil society to enact or sustain a polity,[11] (2) basic procedures sanctioned by the polis, and (3) a common ideal that integrates the first and second values. In a deeply pluralistic state, neither the founding values nor the integrative ideal will be very robust. But that does not prevent them from being powerful. The power of these values, we will find, resides not merely in the fact that the state backs them, but also in the way individuals relate this thin repertoire of common values to their various and diverging thick moralities.

The common values that cause civil society to enact or sustain a polity include the desires for security and liberty, and the resolve to cooperate with others for ends that cannot be attained without cooperation. Persons lacking the latter value may live within the polity, but they are moral outsiders—without legitimate moral claims on goods produced through the association (except insofar as these goods come through the labor or expense of the outsiders or through activities that infringe rights of permission extended by the state to outsiders).[12] Though these values are basic and formative, they are diverse and sometimes mutually at odds. Hence, they do not constitute a fundamental moral principle for the polity.

The most basic procedure sanctioned by the polis is deliberation to a modus vivendi, governed by the principle of permission. Though the principle of permission requires interpretation (primarily regarding the qualifications of permission-givers for various decisions and what counts as their property), it mediates other rules and principles without being susceptible to countermand from a higher principle. Hence, the principle of permission can be regarded as the fundamental principle for a pluralistic, democratic polity.

The common ideal binding members of the polity as a secular moral community is that of diverse individuals and communities pursuing their particular (and sometimes diverging) ends freely, securely, and—when the principle of permission is satisfied—sometimes also cooperatively. This is the civic *telos*, or end, that defines civic teleology. As *telos*, the ideal integrates both the basic common values and the basic procedures (especially the fundamental principle) that characterize the polity. It is neither exclusively rule-oriented, nor exclusively outcome-oriented, nor is it an end point that can be reached in time. To the contrary, it is a process through which common values are expressed and realized in the right way (i.e., in accordance with principles and procedures that are themselves valued by citizens of the polity).

The civic *telos* does not change formally in mass casualty medicine, but its manifestations are distinctive in several respects. First, there is no option of noncooperation. By its very nature, MCM is a cooperative venture; it cannot succeed when citizens or groups opt out of crucial activities such as quarantine, evacuation, and public service. Second, MCM allows little time for extensive deliberation or other permission-getting processes. Most of the public deliberation about MCM measures needs to occur *before* the occurrence of a mass casualty event. One of the central objectives of this book is to stimulate such prior deliberation. Third, civic objectives that come to the fore in MCM are predominately negative—that is, they are concerned with avoiding harms rather than attaining fulfillments. Combined, these factors contribute to the high levels of public spirit and unanimity that typify social action in mass casualty events. Moral visions may diverge significantly between various individuals and moral communities, especially with regard to favored fulfillments; but nearly everyone views violent death and epidemic disease as terrible evils. When the battle against such enemies is heated, unlikely alliances prevail.

For the clinician or rescuer at the front lines, the imperative is to connect with the burgeoning public spirit and serve it, yet always to view pressing health and safety concerns in their proper, broader context—as elements of a civic *telos*.

THE APPROACH TO BALANCING INDIVIDUAL INTEREST AND AGGREGATE INTEREST

The frontline clinician, like any other effective public servant, must have a cause and serve it devotedly. This devotion to a social cause goes by many names—fidelity, honor, integrity, even patriotism. I will call it loyalty.

I have argued in the past that loyalty is the fundamental virtue for all clinicians, in every specialty and every situation, and that clinicians' loyalty should ultimately be grounded in the broadest ideal of the community they serve.[13] The fundamental duty is the same, then, in ordinary clinical medicine and mass casualty medicine: loyalty to the civic *telos*. In both cases, the common ideal requires clinicians (among other things) to strike an appropriate balance between service to particular individual and aggregate interests. However, the stark variation in circumstances between OCM and MCM dictates a corresponding difference in the particular features of this balance, manifested in MCM by the tenets of the Rescue Paradigm (RP).

Recall that RP is differentiated by its intense focus on saving lives and minimizing permanent disability, over and against other possibly competing considerations such as tailoring treatment plans to fit with patients' particular preferences and ideas about the good life. Clinicians operating under RP will depend more on treatment protocols and efficiency-promoting procedures such as disaster triage, and they will consider collective aims such as aggregate survival more prominently in their clinical decision making.

How, then, should the clinician serving in a mass casualty event strike a new and appropriate balance between individual interest and aggregate interest? As we have observed, these two species of interest are not inherently at odds and tend to be aligned more uniformly in MCM than in OCM. But they will nonetheless diverge in some instances, especially in decisions about coercion, where crucial liberty interests of individuals may clash with the aggregate security interest. We also observed that the means of striking an appropriate balance in such decisions will be the proper exercise of practical judgment. Practical judgment is not a deductive affair in which moral principles are applied like recipes to produce distinct and singularly correct solutions. If we are to provide guidance for the cultivation of practical judgment, the best we can do is provide guiding principles or training regimens.

In what follows, I will present eight practical ethical guidelines that build on our earlier discussion. These should, of course, be understood as supplemental to prior conclusions about proper training and the construction of evidence-based practice guidelines. Though they are more precise and focused than the general guidance about loyalty to the *telos*, they nevertheless underdetermine most decisions. Clinicians will not be able to escape the necessity of negotiating gray areas. These guidelines are specifications of loyalty to the civic *telos*, applying in contexts where coercive decisions are at issue.

1. Use all the available information

Decisional guidelines for triage and other clinical procedures in MCM are typically and justifiably based on the assumption that clinicians will be working under pressing time constraints and will have limited information about particular patients (such as social history, tendency to comply with medical instructions, etc.). However, not all decisions in MCM are time constrained, and sometimes clinicians will possess, or have the opportunity to acquire, quite a bit of information about individual patients. In such circumstances, the clinician is obliged to use the additional information. For instance, in the Dr. Adams scenario, the clinician may ascertain that his patient is highly reliable, public-spirited, and inclined to strictly adhere to an at-home quarantine. This information could justifiably tip the decisional scales toward placement in category three.

2. Resolve gaping uncertainties in the direction of major security concerns

As with the Dr. Adams scenario, clinical uncertainty pervades most treatment decisions in MCM. When there is major uncertainty about the clinical outcome of various treatment or triage options, clinicians should be careful not to choose an option that could produce serious harm to the general public. Consider a scenario in which a patient has been exposed to a very contagious, incurable illness such as smallpox and exhibits a noncompliant stance toward restrictive public health measures (the patient, for example, may have refused to cooperate with a tuberculosis treatment program or refused to discontinue unprotected sexual contact with unwitting partners after a diagnosis of AIDS). Assume also that the smallpox outbreak in question has been quickly contained, so that the prospects of preventing an epidemic are good. In such a case, there is major uncertainty about the public risk that would pertain if such a patient were placed in voluntary quarantine—and possibly catastrophic results if the patient failed to cooperate. These considerations might justify placing the patient under supervised enforced quarantine, even if the general presumption in that jurisdiction favored voluntary measures.

3. Do not sacrifice basic liberties for minor security concerns or ineffective interventions

Perhaps this guideline seems so patently obvious that it hardly bears formal iteration. However, it is frequently and egregiously disregarded—often by clinicians and rescuers afflicted by the rescuer's conceit. The rescuer's conceit is a hysterical fantasy that afflicts disaster workers who (1) habitually magnify the importance of their individual decisions, (2) overestimate their personal expertise and moral fortitude relative to ordinary citizens and other rescuers whom they hold morally suspect, (3) self-righteously insist that their authority should be accepted without objections, and hence, (4) feel a measure of delight in enacting coercive measures insofar as it constitutes a kind of vindication of their importance, expertise, moral superiority and authority. This dynamic operates in the aforementioned incident commander who leaps at the opportunity to confiscate hotel property for showering contaminated victims, despite the minimal hazards these victims suffer or pose for others and the sufficiency of alternative noncoercive means of decontamination. And it pertains when clinicians quickly strip nonthreatening victims of their liberties (for instance, by placing relatively noncontagious patients in isolation) on the basis of exaggerated self-congratulatory feelings of being the public's protector. The antidote is a dose of humility—a virtue that cannot be encoded in MCM guidelines but that constitutes a major element of effective practical judgment in all legitimate decisions about coercion.

4. Do not allow suspicion to become a self-fulfilling prophecy

To some degree, clinicians are obliged to be cautious about trusting patients to comply with public safety measures—especially when much is at stake. The general disregard of safe-driving measures is testament to the prevalence of dangerously selfish (or ignorant) attitudes in our population. However, in a mass casualty event, public spirit typically magnifies, as does the perception of a tangible danger, such that willing, intelligent cooperation becomes more likely. As I have argued, this development can be harnessed and appropriated for the public good. But it is also easily extinguished when officials and clinicians exhibit heavy-handedness and general distrust toward the public. In this regard, it is illustrative that quarantine for SARS was more effective in Canada, where citizens were typically viewed as trustworthy allies capable of sustaining voluntary quarantines, than in China, where they were quickly subjected to involuntary measures based on the assumption that they would not cooperate. It is unsurprising that in China patients exposed to SARS were far more apt to flee their cities, spreading contagion to remote areas. Individual clinicians can enhance public cooperation and the effectiveness of MCM measures by treating patients as allies rather than suspects.

5. *Never enact coercive measures when less-coercive measures are sufficient*

This theme runs through much of the guidance already offered. It is imperative that all clinicians and other officials constantly consider noncoercive options, even when a coercive option is the most obvious or the easiest (logistically, the latter will rarely be the case). A noncoercive intervention is sufficient to the task when it is effective in achieving the given public health objective and it will not seriously impede other essential MCM activities.

6. *Avoid mythological thinking*

Again, much of the preceding analysis is predicated on this guidance. The panic myth, for instance, is a prevalent remediable cause of illegitimate uses of coercion. Further illustrations are hardly needed at this point.

7. *Internalize public decisional norms*

Recall the case of Dr. Marcia Welby from the first chapter. Dr. Welby isolated a presumably noncontagious patient because she (rightly) believed it would enhance that patient's chances of surviving the event. Her decision reflected her belief that as a clinician serving in a potential mass casualty event she should do everything in her power to maximize survival. But that was not the intent of legislators who endowed her with the emergency powers. Their intent was to empower her to detain individuals who would otherwise pose a serious health risk to *other citizens*. Dr. Welby failed ethically in this case because she failed to internalize and manifest the ethical content of the public decisional norm she ostensibly enacted. In essence, she forcibly inflicted her own moral vision against the will of the patient and against the will of the public authorities. If one accepts the modus vivendi approach to public deliberation and the recommendation that ethical standards be kept as local as efficiency and logistics allow, then it is inevitable that particular legal and ethical norms for measures such as isolation, quarantine, takings, conscription, mandatory examination, and such will vary between jurisdictions. It is ethically incumbent on rescuers and clinicians serving in a particular jurisdiction to understand the ethical norms that structure MCM in that jurisdiction and to manifest them so far as they are able. Not to heed this obligation is to inflict one's own ethics—by force in the case of coercive decisions.

CONCLUSION: DEALING WITH THE RESCUER'S PARADOX

Loyalty is effective as an ethical orientation just because it integrates intensely personal elements with broadly social ones and does this in a very practical way. Josiah Royce defined loyalty as "the willing and practical and thoroughgoing devotion of a person to a cause."[14] As I observed, for clinicians and other rescuers who serve in MCM, the cause is the civic *telos*. To serve the civic *telos* in an authentic spirit of loyalty, one must embrace it closely—as a matter of deep devotion and as something valuable enough to warrant self-sacrifice. Abstract, scholarly characterizations of the *telos* such as I have offered in this chapter are hardly sufficient to engender such devotion. Anyone who expects to serve this public end must reach beyond austere formulations and connect it to deeply held convictions. Public service must be engrafted into the moral vision; and in times of dire public emergency, it must rise to the fore—emotionally, intellectually, and volitionally.

We might say that the loyal rescuer manifests a deeply felt *love* for the community he or she serves. Such love often remains mostly hidden in day-to-day social interactions, where other matters and other causes garner most of the attention. But if it does not emerge amid the arduous and horrific circumstances of a mass casualty event, then it seems unlikely that clinicians and other rescuers will be able to muster adequate resolve.

The rescuer's devotion to the community is not merely love for the social whole, abstracted from its particular content. Such abstract love is hardly an effective motive, and even less potent as a source of practical judgment in decisions that seriously affect individual persons. To be practical in the way that authentic loyalty is always practical, the rescuer must find the *telos* manifest in the seemingly chaotic admixture of human actions, feelings, strivings, rewards, tragedies, disappointments, and ideals.

At the same time, however, rescuers must strive for a high degree of appropriate objectivity and detachment. As any emergency physician or paramedic can attest, it is impossible to undertake a difficult or intricate procedure while attending to the suffering of the particular patient. One must focus intently on the task at hand. In mass casualty medicine, where suffering and uncertainty (and possibly also personal danger) are prevalent and unrelenting, objectivity and detachment become even more crucial. Without objectivity, burnout and other psychological malfunctions are inevitable and quick.

The contraposition of imperatives for engagement with imperatives for detachment is what I call "the Rescuer's Paradox." It presents a central problem for all persons who work in high-adrenaline, crisis-oriented, cooperative professions. Many who will serve in MCM (emergency physicians, firefighters, battle-tested soldiers, etc.) have professional experience in navigating it. Practical judgment in such professions involves not merely doing the right thing, at the right time, with the right people, in the right way. It also manifests (as Aristotle observed) the right feelings in the right contexts. The transitions between engagement and detachment typically are not abrupt, but more often exhibit the character of musical counterpoint, where each element crescendos as the other fades, all the while relying on its counterpart for proper sustenance and effect.

Earlier, I recommended that states adopt the radical tolerance of indifference. In concluding, I urge readers never to mistake this political doctrine for a virtue of the citizens who acknowledge it. The radical tolerance of indifference is designed to ensure voluntary and peaceful engagement between citizens, not to preclude engagement or to recommend detachment. Crises such as mass casualty events reset the conditions of engagement—compelling citizens to collaborate and sometimes even, through coercion, to limit the opportunities for voluntary disassociation. Insofar as it is possible, citizens should cultivate advance agreements about the terms of coercion in such events. But when the event is at hand, success will hinge on the loyalty of leaders and rescuers—and their ability to render the civic *telos* into a common devotion that informs difficult decisions and inspires suffering individuals to view their destinies as linked.

Notes

1. At a secret 1995 international meeting on dangers from chemical, biological, radiological, and nuclear weapons, Bill Patrick described the ease with which terrorists could obtain colonies of deadly bacteria such as those associated with anthrax, plague, and tularemia. With a starter colony of *Francisella tularensis* (the bacterium causing tularemia) and 1,000 augur plates, terrorists could produce 5 liters of infectious material in 36 hours. This goop, Patrick continued, could be mixed in a food blender and strained through cheesecloth to produce a 5 million bacteria per ml solution, then dispersed into the air intake system of a large building with a garden sprayer. According to Patrick, such a strategy could quickly infect half of the people in the World Trade Center. See Judith Miller, Stephen Engelberg, and William Broad, *Germs: Biological Weapons and America's Secret War* (New York: Simon & Schuster, 2001), 163.

2. Lawrence O. Gostin et al., "The Model State Emergency Health Powers Act: Planning for and Response to Bioterrorism and Naturally Occurring Infectious Diseases," *JAMA* 288, no. 5 (2002): 622–28.

3. The most substantial amendment to the Delaware bill was the second one, in which several of the provisions from MSEHPA were removed. The legislative history of this bill can be reviewed at www.legis.state.de.us/.

4. A "public health emergency" is defined in Section 104, article m, of MSEHPA as "an occurrence or imminent threat of an illness or health condition that: (1) is believed to be caused by any of the following: (i) bioterrorism; (ii) the appearance of a novel or previously controlled or eradicated infectious agent or biological toxin; (iii) [a natural disaster;] (iv) [a chemical attack or accidental release; or] (v) [a nuclear attack or accident]; and (2) poses a high probability of any of the following harms: (i) a large number of deaths in the affected population; (ii) a large number of serious or long-term disabilities in the affected population; (iii) widespread exposure to an infectious or toxic agent that poses a significant risk of substantial future harm to a large number of people in the affected population." This definition has been criticized for the vagueness of terms such as "imminent threat," "high probability," and "large number of deaths"—critics worrying that almost anything could be construed as a public health emergency and thus used as a rationale for instituting highly coercive public health interventions. In defense of the MSEHPA authors, it is generally better to leave a little wiggle room, where personal judgment can operate, than to try to determine action guides too precisely.

What is more concerning to me than the vagueness of the definition of "public health emergency" is the lack of accountability of those applying it. In Section 804, MSEHPA provides that governors and other public health authorities will not be held liable for actions under MSEHPA except in cases of "gross negligence or willful misconduct." In my opinion, any negligence—"gross" or otherwise—should be scrutinized and, where appropriate, punished.

5. David T. Dennis et al., "Tularemia as a Biological Weapon," in *Bioterrorism: Guidelines for Medical and Public Health Management*, ed. Donald A. Henderson, Thomas V. Ingelsby, and Tara O'Toole (Chicago: AMA Press, 2002), 180. The Soviets are known to have produced a vaccine-resistant strain of tularemia. See Ken Alibek and Stephen Handelman, *Biohazard* (New York: Delta, 1999), 25–28.

6. Doxycycline is contraindicated in children less than 9 years old due to tooth enamel hypoplasia (poor growth) and dental staining. It can also cause severe exacerbation of hepatic disease. Ciprofloxacin causes joint disease in immature animals, but this effect is rarely seen in human children. The American Academy of Pediatrics considers ciprofloxacin to be "usually compatible with breastfeeding." See American Academy of Pediatrics Committee on Drugs, "The Transfer of Drugs and Other Chemicals into Human Milk," *Pediatrics* 108, no. 3 (2001): 776–89.

7. Dennis et al., "Tularemia as a Biological Weapon," 169.

8. Many of the American founders subscribed to variations of the Lockean view that persons form political society on the basis of a compact that attenuates certain natural liberties primarily to protect highly vulnerable liberties (freedom from aggression, freedom of conscience, freedom of exchange). See John Locke, *Two Treatises of Government*, ed. Peter Laslett, *Cambridge Texts in the History of Political Thought* (New York: Cambridge University Press, 1988), 350–51. See also Gary Rosen, *American Compact: James Madison and the Problem of the Founding* (Lawrence: University Press of Kansas, 1999), 10–38.

9. Brian D. Mahoney, "Disaster Medical Services," in *Emergency Medicine: A Comprehensive Study Guide*, ed. Judith E Tintinalli, Ernest Ruiz, and Ronald L. Krome (New York: McGraw-Hill, 1996), 20–25.

10. C. E. Fritz, "Disasters," in *Contemporary Social Problems*, ed. R. K. Merton and R. A. Nisbet (New York: Harcourt, 1961), 655.

11. E. L. Quarantelli, *Catastrophes Are Different from Disasters: Some Implications for Crisis Planning and Managing Drawn from Katrina* (Disaster Research Center, 2005). Available online at http://understandingkatrina.ssrc.org/Quarantelli/ [accessed October 28, 2005]. Another aspect of catastrophes, according to Quarantelli, is that the "mass media system especially in recent times socially constructs catastrophes even more than they do disasters." One of the ways in which news media distort reality in catastrophes is by diffusing even more rumors than in disasters. With regard to Hurricane Katrina, Quarantelli writes: "While looting did occur, which is atypical for disasters, the anti-social behavior was widely depicted as typical when the prosocial behavior was by far the norm (it should be noted that a catastrophic situation is only one condition necessary to have mass looting)." Most of the typical false dogmas were also amplified in media coverage of Katrina. For instance, Quarantelli notes, "The question of 'who is in charge' was reiterated over and over again, as if it was a meaningful question, reflecting the command and control model that disaster research has indicated does not work well in disasters, much less in catastrophes."

12. Ibid. Disaster researchers also sometimes differentiate between consensus-type disasters, produced by accidents and nature, and conflict-type disasters, where the harm is intentional. The degree of divergence between these two types of disaster is not well worked out. Though this book focuses somewhat more on conflict-type disasters, both types are under scrutiny. The bulk of disaster research deals with consensus-type disasters, and I draw extensively from such research.

13. My account here conflicts with accounts of disease based on species normal function. See, for instance, Norman Daniels, *Just Health Care*, ed. Daniel I. Wikler, *Studies in Philosophy and Health Policy* (New York: Cambridge University Press, 1985), 28–32. I have argued elsewhere that these latter are untenable, but this issue is somewhat beside the point in the current study. See Griffin Trotter, *The Loyal Physician: Roycean Ethics and the Practice of Medicine*, Vanderbilt Library of American Philosophy (Nashville, Tenn.: Vanderbilt University Press, 1997), 139–41.

14. Griffin Trotter, "Loyalty in the Trenches: Practical Teleology for Office Clinicians Responding to Terrorism," *Journal of Medicine and Philosophy* 29, no. 4 (2004): 390.

15. Eric Auf der Heide, "Common Misconceptions about Disasters: Panic, the 'Disaster Syndrome,' and Looting," in *The First 72 Hours: A Community Approach to Disaster Preparedness*, ed. Margaret O'Leary (New York: iUniverse, 2004).

16. Tom L. Beauchamp and James F. Childress, *Principles of Biomedical Ethics*, 5th ed. (New York: Oxford University Press, 2001), 94–95.

17. Robert Nozick, "Coercion," in *Philosophy, Science, and Method: Essays in Honor of Ernst Nagel*, ed. Sidney Morgenbesser, Patrick Suppes, and Morton White (New York: St. Martin's Press, 1969), 440–72. Bernard Gert, "Coercion and Freedom," in *Coercion: Nomos Xiv*, ed. J. Roland Pennock and John W. Chapman (Chicago: Aldine, Atherton Inc., 1972), 36–37.

18. Beauchamp and Childress, *Principles of Biomedical Ethics*, 94.

19. Nozick would disagree here, since he believes that liberty is not infringed when coercive threats are not credible ("Coercion," 440). But for Beauchamp and Childress (and for me), to count as coercion a threat must be credible—that is, the threatening party will actually carry out the threat.

20. Thomas Hobbes, *Leviathan*, ed. Richard Tuck, *Cambridge Texts in the History of Political Thought* (New York: Cambridge University Press, 1996), 145. Following this lead, John Locke characterized "natural liberty" as the absence of restraints other than the Law of Nature, and "liberty in society" as the absence of restraints other than the Law of Nature and the laws established by a legislative authority to which the subject consents. See Locke, *Two Treatises of Government*, 283–84. We will regard liberty as natural liberty. Thus, in the terminology of this text, infringements of liberty established by a legitimate legislative authority (i.e., an authority established through consent) will still be regarded as infringements, even if they are legitimate ones. This usage will help us remain consonant with the current habit of speaking about legitimate tradeoffs between liberty and other rights or goods.

21. For Hobbes and some other early commentators on the nature of liberty, the category of "external impediments" is sometimes restricted to physical influences that directly impede action. Hobbes believes that "a man sometimes pays his debt, only for *feare* of Imprisonment, which because no body hindred [*sic*] him from detaining, was the action of a man at *liberty*" (*Leviathan*, 146; italics in the Cambridge text).

22. Gert, "Coercion and Freedom."

23. Willard Gaylin and Bruce Jennings, *The Perversion of Autonomy: Coercion and Constraint in Liberal Society*, rev. and exp. ed. (Washington, D.C.: Georgetown University Press, 2003), 144.

24. Ibid., 148.

25. Interestingly, in consulting *Black's Law Dictionary*, Gaylin and Jennings document two legal senses of coercion—one occurring in an "actual, direct or positive" way, "as where physical force is used to compel an action against one's will." Black's second sense of coercion is described as "implied, legal or constructive, as where one party is *constrained* by subjugation to the other to do what his free will would refuse" (italics mine). Black's, then, uses "constraint" to describe coercion's less physical polarity, just the opposite of what Gaylin and Jennings choose to do (ibid., 143).

26. As of this writing, there have been three TopOff exercises (two of these will be discussed later). Another major exercise was Dark Winter, which involved a hypothetical smallpox attack on Oklahoma City. See Tara O'Toole, Michael Mair, and Thomas V. Ingelsby, "Shining Light on 'Dark Winter,'" *Clinical Infectious Diseases* 34 (2002): 972–83.

27. Democrat Tom Huntley, a representative in Minnesota's statehouse, complained, for instance, that "someone with smallpox could walk out of the hospital and nobody could do anything about it." See Sarah Lueck, "States Seek to Strengthen Emergency Powers," *Wall Street Journal*, 7 January 2002.

28. Gostin et al., "Model State Emergency Health Powers Act."

29. The phrase "in collaboration with" appears on the title page of the first draft of MSEHPA but is changed to "to assist" in the second draft, which also contains a disclaimer stating that the "language and content of this draft . . . do not represent the official policy, endorsement, or views of the *Center for Law and the Public's Health*, the CDC, NGA, NCSL, ASTHO, NACCHO, or NAAG, or other governmental or private agencies, departments, institutions, or organizations which have provided funding or guidance." In a letter to George Annas, dated December 28, 2001, CDC director Jeffrey Koplan wrote: "The draft model act does not represent any official or unofficial CDC position." See George Annas, "Terrorism and Human Rights," in *In the Wake of Terror: Medicine and Morality in a Time of Crisis*, ed. Jonathan D. Moreno (Cambridge: MIT Press, 2003), 41–42. Nevertheless, in an article explicating the second draft, published in JAMA in August of 2002, Lawrence Gostin and other architects of the model act claim that the act was drafted "in collaboration with members of national organizations representing governors, legislators, attorneys general, and health commissioners." See Gostin et al., "Model State Emergency Health Powers Act," 622.

30. AIDS activists were concerned that the definition of a public health emergency might encompass patients with HIV infection, thus leading to isolation and quarantine. This problem was fixed in the second draft. Privacy advocates also took alarm, but they received fewer concessions. See Lueck, "States Seek to Strengthen Emergency Powers." In response to brisk criticism, in the second draft the authors eliminated criminal penalties for citizens and physicians who refused to cooperate (though other forms of inducement were substituted).

31. Center for Law and the Public's Health at Georgetown and Johns Hopkins Universities, *The Model State Emergency Health Powers Act* (2001 [accessed April 10, 2002]); available from www.publichealthlaw.net/MSEHPA/MSEHPA2.pdf.

32. By August 11, 2003, 33 states and the District of Columbia had passed bills containing provisions that reflected the content of MSEHPA. This tally includes only legislation passed subsequent to MSEHPA, not existing state powers laws. See Center for Law and the Public's Health at Georgetown and Johns Hopkins Universities, *The Model State Emergency Health Powers Act State Legislative Activity* (2003 [accessed February 15, 2004]); available from www.publichealthlaw.net/Resources/Modellaws.htm.

33. Criteria for interpreting "reasonably suspects" and "endanger the public's health" are not provided in the model act.

34. Coercive isolation and quarantine require a written directive and, within 10 days, a court petition. A hearing will be held within 5 days of the filing of the petition (continued up to 10 days at the court's discretion), authorizing up to 30 days of isolation and quarantine at a time. Subject individuals and groups can challenge isolation and quarantine orders, either by applying to the trial court for an order to show cause why they should not be released (this must be ruled upon within 48 hours), or to request a hearing for remedies regarding breaches to the conditions of isolation and quarantine (hearing date will be fixed within 24 hours when extraordinary circumstances are alleged, or otherwise within 5 days). All individuals and groups subjected to isolation or quarantine will have court appointed legal counsel (Section 605).

35. As the final draft of this book was being put together, the genome for the 1918 avian flu virus was released to the public, stimulating much controversy.

36. George Annas, "Bioterrorism, Public Health, and Civil Liberties," *New England Journal of Medicine* 346, no. 17 (2002): 1338–39.

37. Ibid., 1340.

38. John M. Colmers and Daniel M. Fox, "The Politics of Emergency Health Powers and the Isolation of Public Health," *American Journal of Public Health* 93, no. 3 (2003): 397–99.

39. Mark A. Hall, "The Importance of Trust for Ethics, Law, and Public Policy," *Cambridge Quarterly of Healthcare Ethics* 14, no. 2 (2005): 156–67.

40. Hall actually calls this the "skeptical stance," but I have changed the terminology to underscore Hall's notion that when trust is repudiated, other institutions are substituted to fulfill roles that trust would play, were it operative.

CHAPTER 2: PUBLIC HEALTH AND ITS ETHICAL BASIS

1. Institute of Medicine, *The Future of Public Health* (Washington, D.C.: National Academy Press, 1988). The IOM definition is widely endorsed and frequently cited. See Lawrence O. Gostin, "Tradition, Profession, and Values in Public Health," in *Ethics and Public Health: Model Curriculum*, ed. Bruce Jennings, et al. (Association of Schools of Public Health [Online Publication available at www.asph.org/UserFiles/Module.pdf], 2003), 13. See also James C. Thomas et al., "A Code of Ethics for Public Health," *American Journal of Public Health* 92, no. 7 (2002): 1058.

2. For a rather extreme contrast, compare the levels of physical conditioning required for the "good life" of eighteenth-century Southwest Apaches to those required for the "good life" of twentieth-century accountants.

3. Amitai Etzioni et al., "Communitarian Dialogue: Public Health in the Age of Bioterrorism," *The Responsive Community* 12, no. 2 (2002): 59.

4. Lawrence O. Gostin, "Public Health Law in an Age of Terrorism: Rethinking Individual Rights and Common Goods," *Health Affairs* 21, no. 6 (2002): 80. The call for a new equilibrium between individual and group interests is also prominent in the news media. See, for instance, Nicholas D. Kristof, "Lock 'Em Up," *New York Times*, 2 May 2003. Kristof argues that civil liberties need to be attenuated in deference to law enforcement measures that enhance security against terrorism.

5. Griffin Trotter, "Bioethics and Healthcare Reform: A Whig Response to Weak Consensus," *Cambridge Quarterly of Healthcare Ethics* 11, no. 1 (2002): 45.

6. John Stuart Mill is the classic example. Like most other classical utilitarians, he was a hedonist, defining happiness as pleasure and the absence of pain. See John Stuart Mill, *Utilitarianism*, ed. George Sher (Indianapolis: Hackett, 1979), 7.

7. As egalitarian Amartya Sen notes, "egalitarian" can be applied in a variety of ways, depending on what form of equality one endorses. In general, I will take the term to denote the view that the polis ought to cultivate a robust equality of resources, capacities, or other similar building blocks of the good life, through taxation or other coercive redistributive measures. See Amartya Sen, *Inequality Reexamined* (Cambridge: Harvard University Press, 1992), 12–30. For an analysis of egalitarian trends in pragmatic bioethics, see Griffin Trotter, "Pragmatic Bioethics and the Big Fat Moral Community," *Journal of Medicine and Philosophy* 28, nos. 5–6 (2003): 655–71.

8. Robert N. Bellah, "Community Properly Understood: A Defense of 'Democratic Communitarianism,'" in *The Essential Communitarian Reader*, ed. Amitai Etzioni (Lanham, Md.: Rowman and Littlefield, 1998); Josiah Royce, *The Problem of Christianity*, ed. John J. McDermott (Chicago: University of Chicago Press, 1968).

9. Ezekiel J. Emanuel, *The Ends of Human Life: Medical Ethics in a Liberal Polity* (Cambridge: Harvard University Press, 1991), Griffin Trotter, "Balancing Pluralism and the Common Good: A Look at Open-Air Experiments of Biowarfare Agents," *Accountability in Research* 10 (2003): 109–21.

10. John Rawls, *A Theory of Justice* (Cambridge: Belknap Press of Harvard University Press, 1971), 246.

11. "Primary goods" are defined as "things that every rational man is presumed to want." Rawls's initial broad inventory of primary goods that are "at the disposition of society" includes: "rights and liberties, powers and opportunities, income and wealth" (ibid., 62). This inventory is inconsistent with a conditions model of the common good because it contains elements (such as certain positive rights, certain powers, and income and wealth) that are: (1) desired in widely varying degrees and sometimes not at all (there are ascetics, for instance, who desire neither income nor wealth); (2) interpreted and ranked in radically differing ways, depending on divergent conceptions of the good life; and (3) regarded by some thinkers as things that should not be at the disposition of society. For these reasons, a true conditions model of the common good would focus on conditions that allow for the pursuit of various levels of wealth, income, or capacity—not a state that guarantees the fulfillment of particular wealth, income, or capacity ideals. In defense of his theory, Rawls offers moral assessments that are radically at odds with the commonsense morality of many rational persons. He opines, for instance, that "the idea of rewarding deserts is impracticable," since "the better endowed are more likely, other things being equal, to strive conscientiously" (*A Theory of Justice*, 312). Setting aside the

question-begging qualification (for those who disagree with Rawls, "other things" are morally relevant and they are not equal), Rawls, in importing his intuition that rewards for effort are prima facie unjust, outruns the boundaries of attainable overlapping consensus by several miles.

12. Rawls regards his conception of justice as fairness not as currently enjoying the support of an overlapping consensus, but rather as being a potential object of such consensus over time "in a more or less just constitutional regime, a regime in which the criterion of justice is that political conception itself." In other words, Rawls believes that if we implement his conception of justice by force, then eventually, over the generations, it is possible that the conception can gain the support of an overlapping consensus. See John Rawls, *Political Liberalism* (New York: Columbia University Press, 1996), 15.

13. Alex John London, "Threats to the Common Good: Biochemical Weapons and Human Subjects Research," *Hastings Center Report* 33, no. 5 (2003): 19.

14. Griffin Trotter, *On Royce* (Belmont, Calif.: Wadsworth, 2001), 68–69.

15. London, "Threats to the Common Good," 19.

16. Gostin, "Public Health Law in an Age of Terrorism."

17. The lack of surprise has several sources. First, London's main objective is to show that the corporate conception is an inappropriate way of conceiving the common good in human subjects research settings. It is easier to accomplish this task by pitting it against a double-barreled concept that incorporates both the conditions model and the fulfillment model. Second, distinctions along a continuum (as between the conditions model and the fulfillment model) are more difficult to carry off (though they are almost always more important) than hard-and-fast ones. London had no immediate reason for undertaking this challenge. Third, London's ethical arguments are strongly egalitarian. Like all egalitarians, he derives rhetorical benefits from disguising the connections between his fulfillment model of the common good and its robust underpinnings in a particular moral vision.

18. London, "Threats to the Common Good," 21.

19. Negative rights or classic liberties are rights not to be interfered with. They contrast with positive rights, which are entitlements to goods and services. In our prior discussion of "liberty" (chapter 1), we recognized the possibility of both types of rights.

20. Griffin Trotter, "Emergency Medicine, Terrorism, and Universal Access to Healthcare: A Potent Mixture for Erstwhile Knights-Errant," in *In the Wake of Terror: Medicine and Morality in a Time of Crisis*, ed. Jonathan D. Moreno (Cambridge: MIT Press, 2003), 133–46.

21. Quoted in Daniel Callahan, *What Kind of Life: The Limits of Medical Progress* (New York: Simon and Schuster, 1990), 35.

22. Ibid., 34.

23. Dan E. Beauchamp, *The Health of the Republic: Epidemics, Medicine, and Moralism as Challenges to Democracy* (Philadelphia: Temple University Press, 1988), 98. Another interesting contrast to Beauchamp's view is that expressed by James Madison in his classic treatise on freedom of religion, that the highest duty of citizens is "to take alarm at the first experiment on their liberties" ("Memorial and Remonstrance," in *The Papers of James Madison*, ed. W. T. Hutchinson, W. M. E. Rachal, and Robert A. Rutland [Chicago and Charlottesville: University of Chicago Press and University Press of Virginia, 1962], 299–300).

24. I have seen no evidence supporting the claim that motorcycle helmet laws save money

by reducing medical costs. A study of injury costs associated with motorcycle use in California, comparing costs before and after the enactment of helmet laws, purports to substantiate this claim, but the study is too flawed to be relevant. It does not, for instance, account for the cost of enacting such laws or for the likely shift in motorcycle use away from that state to less regulated states. See W. Max, B. Stark, and S. Root, "Putting a Lid on Injury Costs: The Economic Impact of the California Motorcycle Helmet Law," *Journal of Trauma-Injury, Infection and Critical Care* 45, no. 3 (1998): 550–56. The same flaws have occurred in subsequent studies of the same subject in other states. Of course, not being able to show that helmet non-use is costly does not prove that it isn't costly. In the end, the public cost of not using motorcycle helmets is not highly relevant to the discussion of helmet laws, since there are many means short of coercive helmet laws to ensure that taxpayers and other third parties do not have to pick up the bills. To use cost as a precedent in this case would invite the punishment of far more costly behaviors—casual sex without birth control, for instance—that inevitably tax social and political resources to a much higher degree than riding motorcycles without a helmet does.

25. For a discussion of positivism, its prominence in public health circles, and reasons for being wary of it, see David R. Buchanan, *An Ethic for Health Promotion: Rethinking the Sources of Human Well-Being* (New York: Oxford University Press, 2000), 1–22. For a critique of positivism in the international response to HIV/AIDS, see Griffin Trotter, "Buffalo Eyes: A Take on the Global HIV Epidemic," *Cambridge Quarterly of Healthcare Ethics* 12, no. 4 (2003): 434–43.

26. Griffin Trotter, *The Loyal Physician: Roycean Ethics and the Practice of Medicine*, Vanderbilt Library of American Philosophy (Nashville, Tenn.: Vanderbilt University Press, 1997), 150–51.

27. Ibid., 137–46.

28. H. Tristram Engelhardt Jr., *The Foundations of Bioethics*, 2nd ed. (New York: Oxford University Press, 1996), 199–203.

29. My graduate assistant, Leslie Jumper, searched all issues of the *American Journal of Public Health* from January 2000 to October 2005. During this period, 53 articles addressed the topic of justice (distributive or retributive) in some way. Of these, only 18 make an explicit distributive justice claim. However, most of the articles at least implicitly equate justice with access to health care and public health promotion, often claiming that the purpose of public health interventions is to promote social justice. Only four articles offer a definition of justice, and in two of these the definition is formal (i.e., "justice" is defined by reference to concepts such as "fairness" and "equality" that are as ambiguous as "justice"). Not a single article defends its concept of justice, or its specific justice claims, against competing views.

CHAPTER 3: LEGITIMACY

1. The Germans first used gas on October 27, 1914, in Neuve-Chapelle sector. This attack, using water soluble irritant gases, was ineffective. When they used chlorine gas against the French at Ypres on April 22, 1915, the results were quite different. The green vapor left a four-mile gap with no survivors. Regarding the stigma attached to the introduction of chemical

weapons, Captain B. Liddell Hart's words bear consideration: "The chlorine gas originally used was undeniably cruel, but no worse than the frequent effect of shell or bayonet, and when it was succeeded by improved forms of gas both experience and statistics proved it the least inhumane of modern weapons. But it was novel and therefore labeled an atrocity by a world which condones abuses but detests innovations. Thus Germany incurred the moral odium which inevitably accompanies the use of a novel weapon without any compensating advantage" (*The Real War 1914–1918* [Boston: Little, Brown and Company, 1930], 129–30). Phosgene gas succeeded chlorine and was used by both the Germans and the allies in World War I. It accounted for about 80 percent of the chemical weapons deaths in that war. See Eric Croddy, *Chemical and Biological Warfare* (New York: Copernicus, 2002), 95–96.

2. The by-sea hypothesis was championed by Lieutenant Colonel Philip S. Doane, head of the Health Sanitation Section of the Emergency Fleet Corporation. His thoughts were published by most newspapers and appeared on the front page of the *Philadelphia Inquirer*. See Alfred W. Crosby, *America's Forgotten Pandemic: The Influenza of 1918*, 2nd ed. (New York: Cambridge University Press, 2003), 47.

3. Gina Kolata notes: "If such a plague came today, killing a similar fraction of the U.S. population, 1.5 million Americans would die" (*Flu: The Story of the Great Influenza Pandemic of 1918 and the Search for the Virus That Caused It* [New York: Simon & Schuster, 1999], 7).

4. Crosby, *America's Forgotten Pandemic*, 215.

5. Kolata, *Flu*, 7–8.

6. Crosby, *America's Forgotten Pandemic*, 74–78.

7. Ibid., 92.

8. Ibid., 102–3. The mask ordinance included the following language: "Every person appearing on the public streets, in any public place, or in any assemblage of persons or in any place where two or more persons are congregated, except in homes where only two members of the family are present, and every person engaged in the sale, handling or distribution of foodstuffs or wearing apparel shall wear a mask or covering except when partaking of meals, over the nose and mouth, consisting of four-ply materials known as butter-cloth or fine mesh gauze" (102).

9. Ibid., 104–6.

10. Ibid., 108.

11. Currently there is much fear over the prospect of avian flu, despite a history of apathy about influenza in general (which annually takes thousands of lives). In part, the current concern reflects increased public awareness about the threat of bioterrorism and the recent experience with HIV, with the consequent realization that deadly infectious epidemics are not a thing of the past, even in technologically advanced nations such as the United States. Another factor, however, is the fact that its designation, "avian flu," begets frightening images of dormant evil lurking in exotic natural reservoirs and waiting for export.

12. Mask use may have been somewhat effective in the 1918 epidemic (despite conflicting data). More germane to the activist tendencies of public health authorities (which mirror the same tendencies among physicians in ordinary clinical medicine) is what Crosby has described as the rapid mobilization of virtually every health science institution in the country "to produce with blinding speed absolutely useless vaccines." Immunologically useless vaccines

were pushed avidly by public health authorities such as San Francisco's Hassler, who claimed that, even if they were not effective, the vaccines "cannot do any harm" (Crosby, *America's Forgotten Pandemic*, 313, 100–101).

13. Jürgen Habermas, *Legitimation Crisis*, trans. Thomas McCarthy (Boston: Beacon Press, 1975), 36.

14. James F. Childress et al., "Public Health Ethics: Mapping the Terrain," *Journal of Law, Medicine and Ethics* 30, no. 2 (2002): 173.

15. Ibid., 172. In commenting on a draft of this chapter, H. Tristram Engelhardt Jr. puzzled over the Greenwall scholars' claim that they did not intend their guidelines as universal prescriptions. Engelhardt asked: "Should not all uses of force take into account whether they will be effective, whether they are proportionate, whether they are necessary, etc.?"

16. Ibid., 171.

17. This scenario assumes (as many disaster planners do) that only these two possibilities exist. As we will observe later, there are other preferable alternatives.

18. Michael P. Zuckert, *The Natural Rights Republic* (Notre Dame, Ind.: University of Notre Dame Press, 1996), 49.

19. Joshua Cohen, "Deliberation and Democratic Legitimacy," in *The Good Polity*, ed. Alan Hamlin and Philip Pettit (Oxford: Blackwell Publishers, 1989), 21.

20. A recent book on deliberative democracy contains the following passage: "First-order theories seek to resolve moral disagreement by demonstrating that alternative theories and principles should be rejected. The aim of each is to be the lone theory capable of resolving moral disagreement. The most familiar theories of justice—utilitarianism, libertarianism, liberal egalitarianism, communitarianism—are first-order theories in this sense. . . . In contrast, deliberative democracy is best understood as a second-order theory. Second-order theories are about other theories in the sense that they provide ways of dealing with the claims of conflicting first-order theories. They make room for continuing moral conflict that first-order theories purport to eliminate." (Amy Gutmann and Dennis Thompson, *Why Deliberative Democracy?* [Princeton, N.J.: Princeton University Press, 2004], 13). Though this passage implies that there is only one theory of deliberative democracy, such is not the case. It also seems to imply (wrongly) that second-order theorists do not try to demonstrate that alternative second-order theories should be rejected.

21. Some proponents of RCT would accuse me of overstating their thesis here. Gutmann and Thompson, for instance, have claimed that it is enough if other deliberators can "understand" one's premises—surely a less rigorous requirement than prima facie plausibility as I have described the case. But on closer examination, their use of "understand" seems to imply a hefty dollop of finding something plausible. For instance, they argue that the requirement for submitting only understandable premises precludes deliberators from offering premises drawn or justified from divine revelation. But why would such premises not be understandable? Is "God" really such an obscure concept? If so, why do so many people have an opinion on it? Gutmann and Thompson seem to be arguing that appeals to divine revelation are not acceptable in public deliberation because they invoke beliefs that many will not regard as prima facie plausible (*Why Deliberative Democracy?* 4). In addition, premises drawn from divine revelation are suspect for RCT because they cannot be analyzed by the usual appeals

to science, reason, or collective belief. See Amy Gutmann and Dennis Thompson, *Democracy and Disagreement* (Cambridge: Belknap Press of Harvard University Press, 1996), 55–57.

22. John Rawls, *Political Liberalism* (New York: Columbia University Press, 1996), 144.

23. Incentives to public deliberation have been suggested. Ackerman and Fishkin, for instance, propose a national "Deliberation Day," where all but the most essential work is prohibited by law and all citizens are called to deliberate for a paycheck of $150 "for the day's work of citizenship." Though no one is coerced to deliberate (they are enticed), citizens are certainly coerced into paying for deliberation on this scheme. See Bruce Ackerman and James S. Fishkin, "Deliberation Day," in *Debating Deliberative Democracy*, ed. James S. Fishkin and Peter Laslett (Malden, Mass.: Blackwell Publishing, 2003), 7.

24. Young describes her activist as "committed to social justice and normative value" but leaves it to the reader to sort out what she means by social justice. Her examples of activist opinions make it fairly evident that she intends the concept to be understood in accordance with standard left-wing ideology. Of course, one need not be a leftist to be an activist. To a large extent, right-wing activists (e.g., antiabortion protestors) employ the same cocksure composure and the same aversion to public deliberation and compromise that Young's activist does. See Iris Marion Young, "Activist Challenges to Deliberative Democracy," in *Debating Deliberative Democracy*, ed. James S. Fishkin and Peter Laslett (Malden, Mass.: Blackwell Publishing, 2003), 104.

25. James Madison, "Federalist #10," in *The Federalist Papers*, ed. Clinton Rossiter (New York: Mentor, 1961), 79.

26. Rawls, *Political Liberalism*, 49–50, 164–68. Kurt Baier is cited for his articulation of constitutional consensus.

27. Ibid., 15.

28. It might be objected to my characterization of Hobbes as a proponent of modus vivendi that he was in reality a contractarian—"contractarian" denoting a kind of ethical theory that is closer to being full-fledged than what we find in basic MVT. This objection is correct but also misleading. Hobbes describes "Naturall Lawes" in chapters 14 and 15 of *Leviathan*. His account in these chapters is similar to present-day ideal contract accounts in that it lays out strictures that all men are bound to accept as rational agents on a contractual basis. (Hobbes preferred "nature" to "rationality" but understood nature like most contemporary contractarians understand rationality—in egoistic terms.) The connection with contemporary contractarianism is misleading, on the other hand, because Hobbes refrains from employing an ideal space for negotiation, such as Rawls's original condition or Gauthier's Archimedean point. Hobbes's contract, though ideal, is more a rough, naturally ingrained common prudence than an intricate system of norms that all rational persons are bound to accept. With respect to contemporary contractarians, the ones who import less ethical content into their ideal negotiations are closest to the modus vivendi theorists. Hence, mutual benefit contractarians like Gauthier share much in common with most proponents of MVT. See David Gauthier, *Morals by Agreement* (Oxford: Oxford University Press, 1986).

29. Of course, for Hobbes, the political morality is mostly defined by the will of the sovereign. Our interest in this volume is with democracies. With respect to these latter, John C. Calhoun nicely argues (in a passage we will discuss later) that a unified political view is more

likely to be obtained in a concurrent democracy (where distinctive, incompatible moral communities retain their identity and political power) than in a majoritarian democracy (where they can be easily swallowed). See "A Disquisition on Government," in *Union and Liberty: The Political Philosophy of John C. Calhoun*, ed. Ross M. Lence (Indianapolis: Liberty Fund, 1992), 23–24.

30. George Khushf focuses on another of Locke's reasons for supporting toleration: the limitations of knowledge. The idea here is basically that because reason alone cannot establish a particular conception of the good and the right, we need to tolerate the existence of conceptions that we find wrong or even loathsome. Khushf contrasts this version of toleration with the view maintained by most proponents of rational consensus (who tend to think they have established many of the tenets of the good and the right) that tolerance extends only to practices and beliefs that are compatible with a robust political morality sanctioned by the state. These diverging stances beget two diverging conceptions of pluralism: external pluralism (in which diverging moral communities live according to their particular moral visions) and internal pluralism (in which contrasting lifestyles are allowed but only within the purview of a comprehensive political morality). See George Khushf, "Intolerant Tolerance," *Journal of Medicine and Philosophy* 19 (1994). Modus vivendi theory endorses external pluralism and rejects internal pluralism. Moreover, Khushf's account of Locke's conception of toleration and its rationale is consistent with Hobbes and the thought of several modus vivendi theorists (discussed later in this chapter). Even more than Locke, Hobbes was a moral fallibilist, holding that knowledge is always tentative and hence writing that "no one mans [*sic*] Reason, nor the Reason of any number of men, makes the certaintie" (*Leviathan*, 32). See also Trotter, "Balancing Pluralism and the Common Good," 109–21; and "Bioethics and Healthcare Reform," 44, 50n21, 51n33.

31. Hobbes's sovereign is capable, in theory, of dictating a full-fledged moral doctrine. But this doctrine is not accepted by subjects primarily because it is true or right; it is accepted for prudential reasons that lie at the heart of Hobbes's social contract. In practice, Hobbes's Christian state turns out to be relatively tolerant (as absolute sovereignties go). See Richard E. Flathman, *Thomas Hobbes: Skepticism, Individuality, and Chastened Politics*, ed. Morton Schoolman, New Edition ed., Modernity and Political Thought (Lanham, Md.: Rowman & Littlefield, 2002), 150–55.

32. Hobbes recognizes three fundamental motives for quarrel: (1) competition for material gain, (2) diffidence concerning threats of violence, and (3) desire for glory (*Leviathan*, 88). See also Hobbes's opinions on the "restless desire for power," on hatred as a response to both beneficence and harm, on the preference for sedition over persuasion, on the preference for survival over honor, and on the genesis of credulity from ignorance (*Leviathan*, 70–72, 74). With respect to his emphasis on security from violence, Hobbes is impressed that "the weakest has strength enough to kill the strongest" (*Leviathan*, 87).

33. Patrick Neal, *Liberalism and Its Discontents* (New York: New York University Press, 1997), 192–95.

34. Ibid., 195–97. The italics are Neal's.

35. Even controversies that seem to depend on the most pristinely moral motives are better understood by taking account of other sources of behavior. As sociologist and disaster researcher Benigno E. Aguirre observes, one of the determinants of successful social movements—

especially in time-scarcity cultures—is their ability to integrate the fulfillment of several cultural needs or motives into a compressed period of time. Abortion protestors, for instance, enact civic, ethical, and religious roles simultaneously ("Collective Behavior and Social Movement Theory," in *Disasters, Collective Behavior, and Social Organization*, ed. Russell R. Dynes and Kathleen J. Tierney [Newark: University of Delaware Press, 1994], 258–59). Sociologists have long recognized that rationality and morality are diluted in actual human behavior, though they disagree about the extent of dilution. Expressing one extreme is Randall Collins, who notes the prevalence of the conceit that "pretty much everything we do is based on rational thought processes" but nevertheless holds: "Against all this common sense belief in rationality, however, sociology stands out as a dissenter. One of the central discoveries of sociology is that rationality is limited and appears only under certain conditions. More than that: society itself is ultimately based not upon reasoning or rational agreement but upon a nonrational foundation" (*Sociological Insight* [New York: Oxford University Press, 1982], 3–4). Of course, if rationality and ethics did not pertain in politics or disaster response, there would be no reason for this book. Much sociological research shows that such is not the case. Sometimes, in distinction to the relation specified by Collins, rationality reliably manifests in situations where irrationality is presumed to be the norm. In an article citing the above quotation from Collins, Lewis M. Killian examines this issue. See "Are Social Movements Irrational?" in *Disasters, Collective Behavior, and Social Organization*, ed. Russell R. Dynes and Kathleen J. Tierney (Newark: University of Delaware Press, 1994), 273–80.

36. Stuart Hampshire, *Justice Is Conflict* (Princeton, N.J.: Princeton University Press, 2000), 4.

37. H. Tristram Engelhardt Jr., *The Foundations of Bioethics*, 2nd ed. (New York: Oxford University Press, 1996). Engelhardt's exhaustive treatment of these matters is the best I have seen in the literature of bioethics, political philosophy, or elsewhere. The reader is encouraged to consult it, since Engelhardt argues in far greater detail than the aims of this volume (and the capability of this author) would permit.

38. Hampshire's concept of secular morality (he calls it "liberal morality") is "the rejection of any final and exclusive authority, natural or supernatural, and of the accompanying compulsion and censorship" (*Justice Is Conflict*, 35). Secular morality, for Engelhardt, is the attempt to fashion standards that apply universally—without reference to arbitrary authority. This project begets, on his view, only a procedural morality that tolerates divergent conceptions of the good and right. In his treatise on Christian bioethics, Engelhardt stipulates that "secular" pertains to "moral frameworks that are neutral with respect to religious, including particular, quasi-religious cultural viewpoints." He argues that liberal cosmopolitanism and other ostensibly non-religious or anti-religious perspectives often manifest a quasi-religious character. See H. Tristram Engelhardt Jr., *The Foundations of Christian Bioethics* (Exton, Pa.: Swets & Zeitlinger, 2000), 44, 45n2, 155n35.

39. Engelhardt, *The Foundations of Bioethics*, 69–70. Engelhardt writes: "This view of ethics and bioethics is not grounded in a concern for peaceableness. It is not based on an interest in establishing a peaceable community" (70). This makes him sound terribly non-Hobbesian. For Engelhardt, it is important to clarify that the principle of permission is purely procedural and devoid of content. However, Engelhardt also holds that his procedural principle of secular morality is relevant only to those with an interest "in collaborating with moral

authority in the face of moral disagreements without fundamental recourse to force" (68). Like Hobbes, he regards this interest as inevitable. Unlike Hobbes (and unlike many other modus vivendi theorists, this author included), Engelhardt divorces the motive for secular morality from the justification for its fundamental principle. Engelhardt's conception of a hard-and-fast procedure/substance distinction is debatable and often debated. Hampshire, for instance, argues (to his disappointment): "There is evidently no way of rigorously proving, by an *a priori* argument, that there is an incoherence in not recognising procedural justice as a virtue that is independent of every conception of the good." (Hampshire regards procedural justice in the same way that Engelhardt regards his principle of permission: as the stripped-down requirement for obtaining a legitimate modus vivendi). See Stuart Hampshire, *Innocence and Experience* (Cambridge: Harvard University Press, 1989), 135. Hampshire's point is that any procedure for resolving moral controversies will itself have moral content. Another proponent of modus vivendi, John Gray, concedes the same point (*Two Faces of Liberalism* [New York: New Press, 2000], 25).

40. Hampshire, *Justice Is Conflict*, 41.

41. Ibid., 42.

42. John Gray, *Enlightenment's Wake* (New York: Routledge, 1995), 18–30, Gray, *Two Faces of Liberalism*, 1–33. Gray remarks that today's standard liberal version of tolerance based on the assumption that "one set of liberties is universally legitimate" is illiberal and is, in fact, "a species of fundamentalism, not a remedy for it" (*Two Faces of Liberalism*, 20–21).

43. John Gray mistakenly claims the opposite. See *Two Faces of Liberalism*, 6, 25.

44. Engelhardt, *The Foundations of Bioethics*, 122–23.

45. Engelhardt holds that fetuses, the profoundly mentally retarded, and the hopelessly comatose are examples of humans who are political non-persons (ibid., 138–39).

46. Property rights are constrained, according to Locke, by the qualification that one who appropriates land or resources that he has "mixed with his labor" must leave "enough, and as good" for others. When this qualification is not met, compensation is due. See Locke, *Two Treatises of Government*, 287–88.

47. It would be hard to argue that the ratification of the U.S. Constitution proceeded precisely in accordance with the principle of permission, but within the Federal Convention permission seemed to be the prevailing standard. The Articles of Confederation required unanimity for the enactment of revisions. However, James Madison and several others regarded the Articles of Confederation as a treaty that was null and void due to multiple violations by the states. James Wilson of Pennsylvania argued that the current state of national disarray foisted the delegates into a kind of original position where "the original powers of Society" trumped derivative political rights, and the permission of any state was implied insofar as it refrained from disassociating with the other states. "The house on fire must be extinguished," he said, "without a scrupulous regard to ordinary rights." Though Daniel Carrol and Luther Martin of Maryland argued that 13 votes should be required for ratification, delegates from the other states unanimously rejected this standard. Despite significant contention about the precise requirements, every state other than Maryland agreed in the end that 9 of 13 would be sufficient. In other words, permission was granted for the nine-state standard, and even Maryland seems to have ultimately granted permission by not exercising its prerogative to withdraw. For Madison's views, see James Madison, "Federalist #43," in *The Federalist Papers*,

ed. Clinton Rossiter (New York: Mentor, 1961), 279–80. For the debate about ratification requirements at the Federal Convention, see James Madison, *Notes of Debates in the Federal Convention of 1787 Reported by James Madison*, Bicentennial Edition ed. (New York: W.W. Norton, 1987), 561–65.

48. In matters such as these, Engelhardt's departure from basic MVT is striking, making him look more like deontologically oriented self-ownership libertarian Robert Nozick than like a modus vivendi theorist. No doubt Engelhardt combines elements of both perspectives—and indeed, I have characterized him before as a deontological libertarian when the purpose suited me. To a degree, some kind of overlap between the positions is inevitable. To forge a modus vivendi, there must be negotiators or deliberators, who must in turn be selves or persons—each with ownership of themselves and whatever else they legitimately control. Hence, the terms of ownership must exist prior to deliberation. Yet MVT (in distinction to deontological libertarianism) believes that these terms of ownership are also objects of negotiation and that any particular negotiation will begin where it is (i.e., with whichever constellation of terms of ownership the negotiating parties actually employ). For a self-ownership account of deontological libertarianism, see Robert Nozick, *Anarchy, State, and Utopia* (New York: Basic Books, 1974).

49. Hampshire, *Innocence and Experience*, 11–12, 184–85. Relating how his own moral intuitions arose largely within the context of mid-twentieth-century British politics as a reaction against the British Conservatives, Hampshire disparagingly writes: "For most Conservatives love of property, and of the secure possession of wealth, easily outweighed all other moral commitments" (6). Hampshire's account of an ideal modus vivendi on property would be very different than Engelhardt's.

50. We should acknowledge that rules of property acquisition have changed over the years and that (under the principle of permission) property obtained under one set of rules does not become illegitimate when the rules change—except, of course, when certain types of property are banned outright, as in the socialization of medicine, the banning of guns, or the abolition of slavery. In light of the principle of permission, slaveholders' claims to remuneration for property lost through abolition might seem plausible, were it not for the fact that nonvoluntary slavery itself seems to be the ultimate violation of the principle of permission. If the ownership of other sorts of property, such as medical practices or assault rifles, were banned, then remuneration would surely be in order.

51. Calhoun, "A Disquisition on Government," 30; Engelhardt, *The Foundations of Bioethics*, 116; Gray, *Two Faces of Liberalism*, 116–17; Hampshire, *Innocence and Experience*, 74, 114; James Madison, "Federalist #37," in *The Federalist Papers*, ed. Clinton Rossiter (New York: Mentor, 1961). Much of the this text's discussion of compromise is covered in greater detail in one of my earlier papers: "Bioethics and Healthcare Reform: A Whig Response to Weak Consensus."

52. The new vaccine in this example is a fiction.

53. Weak consensus occurs when a subgroup of inquirers (the "authorized subgroup") internally generates a consensus prescribing behavior for a larger social group (the "target group") that complies but does not share in the consensus. There are three versions of weak consensus, depending on the conditions that cause the target group to acquiesce. In trivial weak consensus, acquiescence is a matter of apathy. In authoritative weak consensus, the tar-

get group complies because they believe on moral grounds that the authorized subgroup should be obeyed. In oligarchic weak consensus, the target population is coerced or otherwise constrained into acquiescence. For a fuller discussion of these phenomena, see Trotter, "Bioethics and Healthcare Reform," 38–42.

54. Calhoun, "A Disquisition on Government," 23–24.

55. Ibid., 30–31.

56. After a very nice discussion of the law of group polarization (a sociological phenomenon in which members of a deliberating group predictably drift toward more extreme versions of the beliefs that polarize them from dissenters), Cass Sunstein advises that we structure political deliberation in a manner that derails polarization and facilitates reasonable conclusions by excluding arguments based on certain divisive beliefs. Which divisive beliefs should be excluded? Sunstein argues that "we often do know enough to know which views count as reasonable, without knowing which view counts as right." Though this statement is certainly true in extreme cases, "our" sense of reasonableness probably lacks sufficient specificity and scope to achieve the kind of consensus-guiding sense that could prescribe "appropriate heterogeneity" (Sunstein's term) without extensive moral imperialism on the part of those designing the deliberative structures. Those whose beliefs are excluded on the basis of someone else's sense of what is reasonable will, in any case, hardly be receptive. See Cass R. Sunstein, "The Law of Group Polarization," in *Debating Deliberative Democracy*, ed. James S. Fishkin and Peter Laslett (Malden, Mass.: Blackwell, 2003). Quotation from page 96.

57. Gutmann and Thompson, *Democracy and Disagreement*, 43, 349–50; Jonathan Moreno, *Deciding Together: Bioethics and Moral Consensus* (New York: Oxford University Press, 1995), 45.

58. The standard practice in clinical ethics, for example, is to initiate consultation with a formal request in which the initiator articulates the particular ethical problem that deliberators are to focus upon. Consensus gurus in bioethics tend to cite John Dewey as one of their intellectual models. Yet even Dewey held that inquiry begins with the identification of a problem and the circumscription of the problem situation. That is not a "common ground" approach.

59. Kevin Wm. Wildes, *Moral Acquaintances: Methodology in Bioethics* (Notre Dame, Ind.: University of Notre Dame Press, 2000), 133.

CHAPTER 4: PUBLIC POLICY AND THE ROLE OF EXPERTS

1. Hugh A. Cowing, "History of the Small-Pox Epidemic at Muncie, Indiana, in 1893," in *Twelfth Annual Report of the State Board of Health of Indiana*, ed. S. S. Boots et al. (Indianapolis: William B. Burford, 1894), 127.

2. Ann E. Mills and Edward M. Spencer, "Evidence-Based Medicine: Why Clinical Ethicists Should Be Concerned," *HEC Forum* 15, no. 3 (2003): 231–44.

3. This emphasis on the use of evidence as medicine's primary ethical imperative is in line with an older habit of viewing technical competence as the primary imperative. See Albert Jonsen's discussion of the ethics of competence in *The New Medicine and the Old Ethics* (Cambridge: Harvard University Press, 1990), 27.

4. Eric Auf der Heide, "The Importance of Evidence-Based Disaster Planning," paper pre-

sented at the Third International WMD Conference, Preparedness through Partnership: Integrating Medical Mass Care Management in a WMD Incident, St. Petersburg, Florida, January 15, 2002.

5. Howard Brody, "Patient Ethics and Evidence-Based Medicine—the Good Healthcare Citizen," *Cambridge Quarterly of Healthcare Ethics* 14, no. 2 (2005): 141–46.

6. Lee Clarke, *Mission Improbable: Using Fantasy Documents to Tame Disaster* (Chicago: University of Chicago Press, 1999), 34–40.

7. Some of the assumptions that guided federal policy include: (1) there will be several days warning before a nuclear attack, giving adequate time to enact evacuations prior to the event (interestingly, Clarke observes that "the rest of the war-making system was premised on thirty minutes' warning, about the time it takes an intercontinental ballistic missile to traverse the northern part of the planet"); (2) there will be adequate food, water, and shelter for evacuees; (3) all evacuees can be protected from radiation; and (4) nuclear targets can be identified in advance. As a contributor to the *Bulletin of the Atomic Scientists* observed, the 80 percent estimate is "an entering assumption, depending on the computer program used to model population evacuation" (ibid., 37). See also Jennifer Leaning and Matthew Leighton, "The World According to FEMA," *Bulletin of the Atomic Scientists* 39 (1983): S2–S6.

8. Clarke, *Mission Improbable*, 37. Italics per Clarke's version. The quoted official is FEMA acting director John W. McConnell, speaking at a hearing before the House Committee on Armed Services, 97th Congress, 1st session, 30 March 1981, p. 4382.

9. Clarke, *Mission Improbable*, 23–30, 84–89.

10. Ibid., 88.

11. H. Tristram Engelhardt Jr., *The Foundations of Bioethics*, 66.

12. Donald A. Henderson et al., "Smallpox as a Biological Weapon," in *Bioterrorism: Guidelines for Medical and Public Health Management*, ed. Donald A. Henderson, Thomas V. Ingelsby, and Tara O'Toole (Chicago: AMA Press, 2002), 105.

13. See Article III, Section 301 of the MSEHPA. Center for Law and the Public's Health at Georgetown and Johns Hopkins Universities, *The Model State Emergency Health Powers Act* (2001 [accessed April 10 2002]); available from www.publichealthlaw.net/MSEHPA/MSEHPA2.pdf. The degree of coercion in such requirements is small—pertaining to the rescission of medical licenses and uses of force that would follow if entities practiced medicine without a license. Such measures amount to minor increases in the intrusiveness of licensing requirements, which are themselves coercive.

14. Bill Frist, *When Every Moment Counts* (Lanham, Md.: Rowman & Littlefield, 2002), 27. Frist's advice coheres with widely disseminated federal guidelines. See Vanessa O'Connell and Nicholas Kulish, "Government Ads Bring More News of Duct Tape and Plastic," *Wall Street Journal*, 19 February 2003. The plastic tape approach has also been used in Israel. Evidently the original source of the U.S. guideline is Ralph E. Comory, president of the Alfred P. Sloan Foundation. See Stephanie Strom, "Behind Duct Tape and Sheeting, an Unlikely Proponent," *New York Times*, 23 February 2003.

15. Strom, "Behind Duct Tape and Sheeting."

16. On March 18, 2003, CNN reported that an Israeli woman and her child suffocated after taping themselves into a bedroom.

17. This recommendation appeared in the committee's June 20, 2002, document "Use of

Smallpox (Vaccinia) Vaccine: Draft Supplemental Recommendation." Previously this document was available online through the Centers for Disease Control (CDC), but as of this writing it is not available online. The recommendation has for the time being been incorporated by the Bush administration into its bioterrorism strategy. See Anonymous, *Protecting Americans: Smallpox Vaccination Program* [Program Statement] (Centers for Disease Control, December 13, 2002 [cited January 8, 2005]); available from www.bt.cdc.gov/agent/smallpox/vaccination/pdf/vaccination-program-statement.pdf.

18. Thomas May and Ross D. Silverman, "Should Smallpox Vaccine Be Made Available to the General Public?" *Kennedy Institute of Ethics Journal* 13, no. 2 (2003): 67–82.

19. Howard Markel, *Quarantine! East European Jewish Immigrants and the New York City Epidemics of 1892* (Baltimore: Johns Hopkins University Press, 1997), 153–65.

20. Griffin Trotter, "Why Were the Benefits of tPA Exaggerated? " *Western Journal of Medicine* 176 (2002): 194–97.

21. I once testified before the U.S. Congress on a bill designed to regulate the reprocessing of single-use medical devices. The drafters of the bill cited only an article from *U.S. News and World Report* as evidence of the problem their bill was designed to address. Unfortunately, the article was highly misleading, containing mostly anecdotal accounts and little useful factual information.

22. Kathleen J. Tierney, Michael K. Lindell, and Ronald W. Perry, *Facing the Unexpected: Disaster Preparedness and Response in the United States* (Washington, D.C.: Joseph Henry Press, 2001), 137–38.

23. E. L. Quarantelli, "Local Mass Media Operations in Disasters in the USA," *Disaster Prevention and Management* 5 (1996): 5–10; E. L. Quarantelli, "Realities and Mythologies in Disaster Films," *Communications: International Journal of Mass Communication Research* 11 (1985): 31–44.

24. E. L. Quarantelli, "The Command Post Point of View in Local Mass Communication Systems," *Communications: International Journal of Mass Communication Research* 7 (1981): 57–73.

25. For surveys of common disaster myths and summaries of the evidence that refutes them, see Eric Auf der Heide, "Common Misconceptions about Disasters: Panic, the 'Disaster Syndrome,' and Looting," in *The First 72 Hours: A Community Approach to Disaster Preparedness,* ed. Margaret O'Leary (New York: iUniverse, 2004), 340–80; Russell R. Dynes, "Disastrous Assumptions About Community Disasters," in *Proceedings of the International Management and Engineering Conference,* ed. James D. Sullivan, Jean Luc Wybo, and Laurent Buisson (Dallas, Tex.: The International Emergency Management and Engineering Society, 1995), 25–28; H. W. Fischer III, *Response to Disaster: Fact Versus Fiction and Its Perpetuation: The Sociology of Disaster* (New York: University Press of America, 1998); E. L. Quarantelli, *How Individuals and Groups React during Disasters: Planning and Managing Implications for EMS Delivery* (University of Delaware, Disaster Research Center, 1989 [cited June 10, 2004]); available from www.udel.edu/DRC/prepapers.html. For a discussion of panic, see E. L. Quarantelli, *The Sociology of Panic* [University of Delaware] (2001 [accessed September 8, 2003]) from www.udel.edu/DRC/preliminary/pp283.pdf. For a discussion of myths about social deterioration during disasters, see Russell R. Dynes, "Finding Order in Disorder: Continuities in the 9–11 Response," *International Journal of Mass Emergencies and Disasters* 21, no. 3 (2003): 9–23.

26. As per the norm, socially adaptive behavior in New Orleans was far more common than antisocial behavior in the aftermath of Katrina. See Quarantelli, *Catastrophes Are Different from Disasters* (Disaster Research Center, 2005). Available from http://understandingkatrina .ssrc.org/Quarantelli/ [accessed October 28, 2005].

27. Jim Dwyer and Christopher Drew, "Fear Exceeded Crime's Reality in New Orleans," *New York Times*, 29 September 2005.

28. Russell Dynes cites several instances of misguided concern about panic, including the headline: "America Is Dangerously Vulnerable to Panic in Terror Attack, Experts Say." See Dynes, "Finding Order in Disorder," 13.

CHAPTER 5: PUBLIC DELIBERATION AND STRATEGIC LEADERSHIP

1. There are certainly exceptions to the generalization that citizens tend to be over-vigorous in their pursuit of safety from nuclear, biological, and chemical terrors. For instance, citizens never really got on board with federal civil defense programs aimed at preparing them to act decisively and adaptively in the event of a nuclear attack. This reluctance seems not so much based on lack of fear of a nuclear holocaust (though toward the end of the Cold War this fear seemed to be waning), but rather on a lack of confidence that the protective meas-ures would work. This lack of confidence hardly seems ill-informed or otherwise indicative of a poor decisional capacity. As Spencer Weart observes, "Even the RAND strategists and local civil defense officials who worked professionally on fallout shelters usually did not build one for their own families" ("History of American Attitudes to Civil Defense," in *Civil Defense: A Choice of Disasters*, ed. John Dowling and Evans M. Harrell [New York: American Institute of Physics, 1987], 25). For a general discussion of this lack of responsiveness to civil defense ini-tiatives, see Lee Clarke, *Mission Improbable*, 117-25.

2. I do not presume to equate moral communities with ideologies. What I do presume is that when moral communities carve a political presence robust enough to be noticed by out-siders, the stable elements of the communities' political input will be regarded (at least by the outsiders) as elements of a political ideology. The term *ideology* has taken on negative conno-tations in recent years, but I am not keen to accentuate these. For present purposes, we should regard a political ideology merely as a nexus of stable beliefs, theories, and habits that consti-tute the core elements of a political program.

3. Many left-liberal political theorists assume that being free to radically modify one's life plan or one's conception of the good (hence, also one's allegiances) is the most fundamental liberty—and that this freedom is meaningless unless the government assures the conditions to enact such modifications successfully. Norman Daniels, for instance, claims that persons have a right to health care insofar as health care is a prerequisite for "normal species functioning." "Normal species functioning" becomes an essentially political category, regarded as funda-mentally important for all persons (even those whose life plans or conceptions of health don't demand Daniels' version of it) because it opens up a range of alternative life plans and, with these, alternative conceptions of the good. Daniels writes: "Consequently, if persons have a fundamental interest in preserving the opportunity to revise their conceptions of the good through time, then they will have a pressing interest in maintaining normal species function-ing . . . by establishing institutions, such as health-care systems, which do just that." Daniels

thinks the state should determine which potential life plans or conceptions of the good are legitimate, then fashion a notion of "normal species function" that potentiates these. The upshot, of course, is that taxpayers are coerced into paying for "options" that some of them find abhorrent or evil, just because the government says they have a fundamental interest in preserving them. See Norman Daniels, *Just Health Care*, ed. Daniel I. Wikler, *Studies in Philosophy and Health Policy* (New York: Cambridge University Press, 1985), 27–28. On the other end of the spectrum, we have theorists like Friedrich von Hayek, who believe that conceptions of the good are in competition and that an important aspect of this competition is the conceptions' relative ability to generate goods and services necessary to sustain those who affirm the conception. On this account, Daniels' big-government approach amounts to a total quashing of legitimate moral pluralism. See Friedrich von Hayek, "Equality, Value, and Merit," in *The Essence of Hayek*, ed. Chiaki Nishiyama and Kurt R. Leube (Stanford, Calif.: Hoover Institution Press, 1984), 32.

4. See Cass R. Sunstein, "The Law of Group Polarization," in *Debating Deliberative Democracy*, ed. James S. Fishkin and Peter Laslett (Malden, Mass.: Blackwell, 2003), 80–101.

5. Bruce Ackerman and James S. Fishkin, "Deliberation Day," in *Debating Deliberative Democracy*, ed. James S. Fishkin and Peter Laslett (Malden, Mass.: Blackwell Publishing, 2003), 7–30. In deliberative polling, "a random sample is first given a survey of the conventional sort. Then it is invited to come to a single place, at the expense of the project, to engage in a weekend of small group discussions and larger plenary sessions in which it is given extensive opportunities to get good information, exchange competing points of view and come to a considered judgment. The resulting changes of opinion are often dramatic. They offer a glimpse of democratic possibilities—the views people would have if they were effectively motivated to pay attention and get good information and discuss the issues together. The Deliberative Poll puts scientific random samples in a situation where they have incentives, in effect, to overcome rational ignorance" (11–12). Deliberation Day is an extension of this sort of program to local, regional, or national politics.

6. Margaret Humphreys, *Yellow Fever and the South* (Baltimore: Johns Hopkins University Press, 1992), 45–76.

7. The term "evidence-based public health" was not used by advocates of the national system or by anyone else in the nineteenth century as far as I know. But the aspirations were clearly there—and not just for public health nationalists. In the 1890s state officials throughout the country pushed for measures that would facilitate data taking. These aspirations were evident, for instance, in public health advocacy for mandatory death permits, burial permits, and public cemeteries. Though many take such measures for granted now, it still is remarkable that the state was able so quickly to usurp control of something so personal and sacred as the handling of dead bodies. See S. S. Boots et al., *Twelfth Annual Report of the State Board of Health of Indiana* (Indianapolis: William B. Burford, 1894), 11–19.

8. Humphreys, *Yellow Fever and the South*, 128–32.

9. George Annas, "Bioterrorism, Public Health, and Civil Liberties," *New England Journal of Medicine* 346, no. 17 (2002): 1340.

10. Calhoun was a prominent antebellum senator (as well as vice president under Andrew Jackson before resigning) and constitutional scholar known for his doctrine of nullification, which holds that states have the right to nullify federal legislation that they find egregiously

unconstitutional. See John C. Calhoun, "The Fort Hill Address: On the Relations of the States and Federal Government (1831)," in *Union and Liberty: The Political Philosophy of John C. Calhoun*, ed. Ross M. Lence (Indianapolis: Liberty Fund, 1992), 370–71.

11. Gary A. Kreps and Susan Lovegren Bosworth, *Organizing, Role Enactment, and Disaster* (Newark: University of Delaware Press, 1994), 99, 154–56, 74–79. As Kreps and Bosworth observe, many intuitively important role linkages have not been studied systematically.

12. Lisa D. Rotz et al., "Public Health Assessment of Potential Biological Weapons," *Emerging Infectious Diseases [on-line]* 8, no. 2 (2002).

13. I do not include threat duration in this classification scheme because, as it turns out, this category doesn't add useful permutations. All of the D_1 and D_2 threats are short duration threats. D_3 threats are a mixed bag, but it turns out that the high-duration ones are also transmissible, so are thus captured on that axis.

14. The ease of disseminating an agent is a related feature that is also of great practical importance. It is not included in this scheme because it is important for terrorists and forensic workers—not to those who must respond after a threat has already been disseminated (except perhaps insofar as they have reason to fear that more agents have been or will be released).

CHAPTER 6: TACTICAL LEADERSHIP

1. Thomas H. Kean et al., *The 9/11 Commission Report: Final Report of the National Commission on Terrorist Attacks Upon the United States*, authorized ed. (New York: W.W. Norton, 2004), 10–14. Subsequent page numbers in the text are from this edition.

2. On United Flight 175, passenger Peter Hanson phoned his father and told him: "I think they've taken over the cockpit—An attendant has been stabbed—and someone else up front may have been killed. The plane is making strange moves. Call United Airlines—Tell them it's Flight 175, Boston to LA." A flight attendant contacted the United office in San Francisco at the same time, reporting that both pilots had been killed and the hijackers were probably flying the plane. Seven minutes later, at 8:59 a.m., Brian David Sweeney called his mother and told her passengers were thinking about storming the cockpit. Unfortunately, that call came only 4 minutes before Flight 175 crashed into the South Tower of the World Trade Center. There were also several informative calls placed from passengers on American Flight 77 (destined to crash into the Pentagon), including two calls to the Solicitor General of the United States from his wife, Barbara Olsen. The Commission reports that, when he informed her of the previous hijackings and crashes, Mrs. Olsen "did not display signs of panic and did not indicate any awareness of an impending crash" (ibid., 7–10).

3. Actually, in the typical mass casualty event, speed to definitive treatment is a *less* important aspect of medical decisions than it is in ordinary emergency medicine. See E. L. Quarantelli, "Converting Disaster Scholarship into Effective Disaster Planning and Managing: Possibilities and Limitations," *International Journal of Mass Emergencies and Disasters* 11, no. 1 (1993): 21.

4. Daniel Henninger, "Leviathan 101: Don't Blame It on FEMA," *Wall Street Journal*, 30 September 2005. Henninger claims that the implicit message from the public denouncement of FEMA director Michael Brown for senior managers in the federal bureaucracy is: "Be careful, not decisive." This message, Henninger thinks, will impede needed internal reforms. He

also comments on the turf battle between DHS and the Pentagon. For an account of another turf battle, between DHS and the Department of Justice, see Robert Block and Gary Fields, "Washington Turf Battle Muddles Nation's Terror-Warning System," *Wall Street Journal*, 28 May 2004.

5. W. A. Lake, P. D. Fedele, and S. M. Marshall, "Guidelines for Mass Casualty Decontamination During a Terrorist Chemical Agent Incident" (Aberdeen Proving Ground, Md.: U.S. Army Soldier and Biological Chemical Command, 2000), 37–38.

6. H. Nozaki et al., "Secondary Exposure of Medical Staff to Sarin Vapor in the Emergency Room," *Intensive Care Medicine* 21 (1995): 1032–35, Sadayoshi Ohbu et al., "Sarin Poisoning on Tokyo Subway," *Southern Medical Journal* 90 (1997): 587–93.

7. Nerve agents such as sarin, tabun, soman, and VX work by inhibiting the enzyme acetyl cholinesterase. This enzyme breaks down the neurotransmitter acetyl choline at the nerve synapse. When acetyl cholinesterase is inhibited, excessive levels of the neurotransmitter accumulate, causing excessive nerve discharge and symptoms such as excessive tearing, salivation, urination, defecation, vomiting, and airway secretion. Pharmacological treatment for nerve agent poisoning must be delivered early or it will be practically useless. In some instances (e.g., military engagements in which the use of nerve agents can be foreseen) pretreatment with carbamates such as pyridostigmine is possible and effective. Two classes of drug are used for treating an established poisoning: (1) muscarinic agents such as atropine that mitigate the effect of excess acetyl choline by blocking receptors at the synapse, and (2) oximes, such as pralidoxime (2-PAM), HI-6, and obidoxim, that reactivate damaged acetyl cholinesterase. See Griffin Trotter, "Chemical Terrorism and the Ethics of Decontamination," *Journal of Clinical Ethics* 15, no. 2 (2004): 149–51.

8. Doctors at Keio University Hospital had advance warning from the metropolitan fire agency that there was "a gas explosion in the Tokyo subway," but no news about chemical casualties. Nozaki et al., "Secondary Exposure of Medical Staff," 1033.

9. Jacek Franaszek, "Is Emergency Department Overcrowding a Disaster?" in *The First 72 Hours*, ed. Margaret O'Leary (New York: iUniverse, 2004), 136–42; Trotter, "Emergency Medicine, Terrorism, and Universal Access to Healthcare," 133–46.

10. "Hazmat" is a contraction for "hazardous materials."

11. Joseph F. Waeckerle, "Domestic Preparedness for Events Involving Weapons of Mass Destruction," *JAMA* 283, no. 2 (2000): 252–54.

12. From the perspective of the frontline medical care provider, the reason that treatment for critically ill, unlikely-to-be-salvaged patients is foregone is because there is limited time and it must be used wisely. So from this perspective, time may well be the primary limiting condition. But from a larger tactical or strategic viewpoint, the real problem is with logistics. There will typically be many providers and plenty of equipment—either somewhere in the community or on their way from elsewhere. How to get these resources properly situated is another matter.

13. Gostin et al., "The Model State Emergency Health Powers Act," 622–28.

14. James Bondi, "School Security and Strategic National Stockpile Distribution Site Operations," in *The First 72 Hours*, ed. Margaret O'Leary (New York: iUniverse, 2004), 67–68.

15. Recently the term "Incident Management System" has begun to circulate. I prefer this term, for reasons that should become obvious. However, I will stick with the older term, "Inci-

dent Command System," because it is more familiar and is the term used in many important documents such as the 9/11 Commission Report.

16. FIRESCOPE is Fire Resources of Southern California Organized for Potential Emergencies. Seven fire agencies, funded by the Federal Emergency Management Agency (FEMA), formed the FIRESCOPE task force that developed the Incident Command System. For a detailed description of the ICS and the related "unified command," see Robert L. Irwin, "The Incident Command System," in *Disaster Response: Principles of Preparation and Coordination*, ed. Eric Auf der Heide (1989).

17. Joe Gasparich, *Biot #9: Introduction to Incident Management* (Lecture from Illinois Bioterrorism Summit, May 28-30, 2002) (Suburban Emergency Management Project (SEMP), 2002 [cited April 28, 2005]); available from www.semp.us.

18. Dennis Wenger, E. L. Quarantelli, and Russell R. Dynes, "Disaster Analysis: Police and Fire Departments, Final Report #1 on Phase II for Federal Emergency Management Agency" (Newark, Del.: Disaster Research Center, 1989), 57–60.

19. Ibid., 156–57.

20. DRC researchers state that the empirical evidence from their studies as well as from their review of the existing literature "indicate that not only are there inherent problems in the 'Incident Command System,' but it can actually contribute to serious difficulties in emergency response." They identify six major problems (most of which we have covered or will cover): (1) the term "Incident Command System" has become more a "buzzword" than a particular detailed management model; (2) the weakest of the elements of the formal ICS—i.e., the "bump up, bump down" command structure—is the one most often adopted; (3) ICS emphasizes intraorganizational planning over interorganizational planning, but the latter is a primary necessity in major disasters; (4) ICS is weak on integrating activities with strategic organizations and with volunteers and/or relief agencies; (5) ICS has problems in disasters that occur in "focused, limited areas," because it tends to bring too many responders and too much congestion to a disaster scene; and (6) the ICS has several internal glitches or limitations that need to be worked out critically—a prospect that seems unlikely where ICS is viewed as a panacea for disaster organization. Since this assessment in 1989, there have been many thoughtful and effective attempts to address most of these difficulties. However, as the term "Incident Command System" has become even more familiar, the concept seems to have become even more diffuse, such that many of the above listed problems are in some jurisdictions even more acute now than they were then (ibid., 156).

21. A California researcher, Dana Cole, recently conducted a "system performance audit" in which 206 California officials were queried about the performance of the Incident Command System in that state. There was a 60 percent response rate, and respondents rated 16 attributes of ICS on a 10-point scale. Cole observes that "despite the emergence of ICS as the world's leading management system for the command, control, and coordination of emergency services, there has never been a comprehensive performance evaluation." Cole's research, though helpful in some respects, hardly counts as such an evaluation. The highest satisfaction ratings in Cole's survey were for "predefined hierarchy" and "uniform terminology" (8.80 and 8.73, respectively). The lowest rankings still reflected significant satisfaction and were received for such notable aspects as "transition of authority" (7.50), "integration of non-fire agencies" (6.84), "integration of non-government" (6.27), and "agreement on system

modifications" (6.23). One of the limitations of this survey is that it involved only relatively high-ranking officials. Their generally high level of satisfaction for items related to establishing their roles as leaders may reflect their place in the hierarchy of authority and their relative insulation from frontline decisions and action.

22. Kean et al., *The 9/11 Commission Report*, 397.

23. In arguing that the EOC is a complex, dynamic social system (and that "no one particular social arrangement or form" is decisively better than the others), Quarantelli remarked in 1997 that liaison officers in the ICS need to be well-informed and vested with significant decisional authority, otherwise their interaction with officials from the various participating organizations will have few practical bearings. E. L. Quarantelli, "Ten Criteria for Evaluating the Management of Community Disasters," *Disasters* 21, no. 1 (1997): 52. Bearing out Quarantelli's advice, the worthlessness of uninformed, unvested liaisons was amply illustrated in 9/11 aerospace defense, as FAA and White House Teleconferences failed to recruit the right officials and therefore produced no meaningful contribution. Kean et al., *The 9/11 Commission Report*, 36–38.

24. E. L. Quarantelli, "The Questionable Nature of the Incident Command System," in *The First 72 Hours*, ed. Margaret O'Leary (New York: iUniverse, 2004), 538–39.

25. Quarantelli, "Ten Criteria for Evaluating the Management of Community Disasters," 50. See also Quarantelli, "The Questionable Nature of the Incident Command System."

26. Wenger, Quarantelli, and Dynes, "Disaster Analysis: Police and Fire Departments," 162.

27. Quarantelli, "Ten Criteria for Evaluating the Management of Community Disasters," 48.

28. Kathleen J. Tierney, Michael K. Lindell, and Ronald W. Perry, *Facing the Unexpected: Disaster Preparedness and Response in the United States* (Washington, D.C.: Joseph Henry Press, 2001), 129.

29. Quarantelli, "Converting Disaster Scholarship into Effective Disaster Planning," 21.

30. EMTALA is the Emergency Medical Treatment and Active Labor Act. Enacted in 1986, it requires that all patients presenting to emergency departments of hospitals that accept Medicare get screened to determine if they have an emergency medical condition. If they do, they must be stabilized before transfer, and certain arrangements need to be made to assure that the transfer is done safely. Most troublesomely to emergency physicians and seriously ill nontransfer patients, who must go untended during the paperwork shuffle, the whole process must be documented in meticulous detail by the transferring physician. A large and daunting bureaucracy has evolved in the monitoring and enforcement of EMTALA, often producing paperwork requirements that have little warrant in the actual legislation. Virtually all disaster plans call for egregious violations of EMTALA—a topic that generated serious concern in the wake of the 9/11 attacks, as planners went into high gear. To ease the anxiety, in the fall of 2001, the Health Care Financing Administration (now the Center for Medicare and Medicaid Services, or CMS) issued a statement on their Web site that EMTALA violations undertaken during the enactment of a disaster plan will not be punished so long as they are "in accordance with" the plan. It is likely that CMS, and some health care providers, will understand "in accordance with the plan" as entailing strict chain-of-command authority. If so, adaptive emergent behavior will be discouraged. For more discussion about EMTALA and its rele-

vance to disaster medicine, see Trotter, "Emergency Medicine, Terrorism, and Universal Access to Healthcare."

31. Recall the fourfold typology employed by the DRC. Type III organizations are called "extending" because "much of what they do is unanticipated." Hospitals functioning in disasters are usually regarded as a prototype of the Type I organization—an "established" organization that neither expands significantly (i.e., by taking on new personnel) nor undertakes unanticipated tasks. However, our example shows how even a Type I organization must deal with unanticipated contingencies (though one would hope that ED overload is not widely unanticipated in contemporary practice)—many of the protocols and practices that address these unanticipated contingencies will be emergent. See Gary A. Kreps and Susan Lovegren Bosworth, *Organizing, Role Enactment, and Disaster* (Newark: University of Delaware Press, 1994), 22–23.

32. I have argued, at book length, that professional loyalties are justified through their grounding in deeper loyalties to the public (and ultimately, to humanity). Griffin Trotter, *The Loyal Physician: Roycean Ethics and the Practice of Medicine* (Nashville, Tenn.: Vanderbilt University Press, 1997). Some of the arguments in that book employ premises that stretch beyond what is likely to be engrafted into the public philosophy of a secular pluralistic society like the United States. But it isn't much of a stretch to claim that "good reasons legitimacy" in a public health emergency will hinge on serving the public, and that anyone who brings harm to another person or abridges their rights, based on idiosyncratic personal and professional values, will (and should) be held blameworthy.

33. For an account of prominent myths regarding preparedness for bioterrorism, see Eric Noji, Tress Goodwin, and Michael Hopmeier, "Demystifying Bioterrorism: Misinformation and Misperceptions," *Prehospital and Disaster Medicine* 20, no. 1 (2005): 3–6.

34. Though extensive experience in multiple disasters is without question likely to be an asset, a little experience may be a liability. Quarantelli notes, for instance, that "success in coping with a past disaster" may be, for the community in question, "more of a disadvantage than not having any experience at all" because it tends to beget the complacency of thinking that the next disaster will be something like the one already experienced. Such complacency may be particularly dangerous in preparations for terrorism, since intelligent terrorists can consciously exploit it. See Quarantelli, "Converting Disaster Scholarship into Effective Disaster Planning," 31.

35. Ibid.

36. The *Journal* reported that on May 12 people would be getting sick with plague in Chicago (the fake terrorists having released it over the weekend at O'Hare and Midway Airports) just as a diversionary dirty bomb detonated in Seattle. The National Strategic Stockpile of drugs would fly in on May 14; the FBI would take down a fake germ lab on May 15; and deaths would mount into the hundreds, casualties into the thousands, by May 16. Marilyn Chase, "Coming Drill Will Simulate Plague Germs in Chicago, Dirty-Bomb in Seattle," *Wall Street Journal*, 2 May 2003.

37. Trotter, "Loyalty in the Trenches," 409.

38. Lake, Fedele, and Marshall, "Guidelines for Mass Casualty Decontamination"; Howard W. Levitin et al., "Decontamination of Mass Casualties—Re-Evaluating Existing Dogma," *Prehospital and Disaster Medicine* 18, no. 3 (2003): 200–207; Henry J. Siegelson,

"Preparing for a Terrorist Attack: Mass Casualty Management," presented at the Third International WMD Conference, St. Petersburg, Florida, January 15, 2002.

39. Underpants may be significantly contaminated in vapor exposures if the victim is wearing outer garments such as a short skirt. Water flushing a patient with contaminated underwear could, in theory, make matters worse by facilitating transdermal absorption.

40. Siegelson, "Preparing for a Terrorist Attack."

41. Quarantelli, "Converting Disaster Scholarship into Effective Disaster Planning," 26. In his discussion of citizens recently increasing demands for involvement in disaster planning, Quarantelli alludes to a law "that requires citizen input into the Corps of Engineering flood planning projects before they are actually initiated."

42. Bureaucratic requirements unquestionably played a role in these limitations. For instance, each volunteer was required to sign a detailed consent form, which included the following: "I understand that as a participant in the mock disaster drill, I may have makeup applied so as to look like a disaster victim; may have my clothing soiled or torn; and may be transported by stretcher [or] wheelchair." See Chase, "Coming Drill Will Simulate Plague."

43. This practice was passed on from TopOff1, where contractors constructed a *Virtual News Network* of actors in black satin jackets "rather than risk interaction with real reporters, a prospect that one participant called as daunting as plague." See Judith Miller, Stephen Engelberg, and William Broad, *Germs: Biological Weapons and America's Secret War* (New York: Simon & Schuster, 2001), 272.

44. Tierney, Lindell, and Perry, *Facing the Unexpected*, 136.

45. Dennis Wenger and E. L. Quarantelli, "Local Mass Media Operations, Problems and Products in Disasters, Report Series #19, University of Delaware Disaster Research Center, 1989, 55–62. (Quotation from page 62). See also: Russell R. Dynes and E. L. Quarantelli, "The Family and Community Context of Individual Reactions to Disaster," in *Emergency and Disaster Management: A Mental Health Sourcebook*, ed. Howard J. Parad, H. L. P. Resnik, and Libbie G. Parad (Bowie, Maryland: Charles Press Publishers, 1976), 231–44.

46. Wenger and Quarantelli, "Local Mass Media Operations, Problems and Products in Disasters," 55. In an article for the *Wall Street Journal*, David Baltimore decries the ways in which fellow journalists create the kind of hysteria that they erroneously assume to be the norm. As an example, Baltimore cites the coverage of the SARS epidemic and how it eventuated in irrational actions such as the boycott of Chinese restaurants ("SAMS—Severe Acute Media Syndrome?" *Wall Street Journal*, 28 April 2003).

47. Kean et al., *The 9/11 Commission Report*, 318.

48. Alan Kaplan, "The Greater Good: The Role of a Hospital Chief Medical Officer in Disasters," in *The First 72 Hours*, ed. Margaret O'Leary (New York: iUniverse, 2004), 62; Wenger, Quarantelli, and Dynes, "Disaster Analysis: Police and Fire Departments," 92, 153. Likewise, the genuine authority that legitimates tactical leaders cannot be assigned or imposed. It is established over time. See Wenger, Quarantelli, and Dynes, "Disaster Analysis: Police and Fire Departments," 134.

49. It is worth noting, however, that role complementarity is not the rule in emergent and extending organizations, and that volunteers and other strangers who come together specifically in a disaster situation commonly work very well together. See Kreps and Bosworth, *Organizing, Role Enactment, and Disaster*, 106, 36, 77.

50. Quarantelli, "Ten Criteria for Evaluating the Management of Community Disasters," 46; Tierney, Lindell, and Perry, *Facing the Unexpected*, 129; Wenger, Quarantelli, and Dynes, "Disaster Analysis: Police and Fire Departments," 147. Even in the aftermath of the 9/11 tragedy, longstanding tensions between the New York City police and fire departments still smolder and forebode problems in future disaster operations. At this writing, one major point of contention is that city planners have designated police officials to take command in a disaster.

51. Quarantelli, "Converting Disaster Scholarship into Effective Disaster Planning," 29.

52. Quarantelli, "Ten Criteria for Evaluating the Management of Community Disasters," 48–49.

53. In cynical moments, I wonder if the bureaucratic mentality typifying so many public officials can ever be effectively adapted to the contingencies of a disaster, and I suppose that the only hope is to appropriate private-sector talent—from industries where adaptive thinking is regarded as an essential asset rather than a dangerous invitation to punitive oversight. In November of 2005, the *Wall Street Journal* published an intriguing article that documented how various private logistics experts assisted in the year's numerous disasters. The lead story featured Chris Weeks, an express shipping executive from DHL Corporation. In the response to a Kashmir earthquake in October 2005, Weeks (who was "on loan" from DHL to the U.S. military) helped devise a "speedball" approach for distributing needed food and supplies to remote sites. The "speedball" was a red polypropylene ball of the sort DHL uses to move loose cargo, on this occasion stuffed with enough food, tents, and other supplies to keep seven people alive for ten days. Thousands of speedballs were distributed by helicopter to difficult-to-reach outposts—helicopters swooping down and the crew kicking them out, then quickly moving on to the next destination. See Glenn R. Simpson, "In Year of Disasters, Experts Bring Order to Chaos of Relief," *Wall Street Journal*, 22 November 2005.

CHAPTER 7: DECISIONS FOR PARTICULAR COERCIVE ACTIONS

1. Margaret Humphreys, *Yellow Fever and the South* (Baltimore: Johns Hopkins University Press, 1992), 61, 138. Also, during the cholera epidemics, the health officer of the Port of New York, Dr. William Jenkins, shipped the wealthier quarantined to Fire Island. Howard Markel reports that "a gaggle of resident clam-diggers tried to prevent these boats from landing with sticks and guns, until New York Gov. Roswell Flowers ordered the National Guard to subdue them" ("Quarantine," *Wall Street Journal*, 7 October 2005.

2. Eric Auf der Heide, "Common Misconceptions About Disasters: Panic, the 'Disaster Syndrome,' and Looting," in *The First 72 Hours: A Community Approach to Disaster Preparedness*, ed. Margaret O'Leary (New York: iUniverse, 2004), 363. (Auf der Heide's citations are omitted from the quotation.)

3. Regarding measures designed to enhance the comfort of public officials who must use force against innocent civilians, consider the provision in the first version of the MSEHPA holding that the right to contest involuntary quarantine will be suspended during weekends and holidays—Section 503(e)(3). One might question the prerogative of public officials presiding over such events to be taking holidays.

4. This scenario was considered in an earlier essay, Griffin Trotter, "Loyalty in the Trenches: Practical Teleology for Office Clinicians Responding to Terrorism," *Journal of Med-*

icine and Philosophy 29, no. 4 (2004): 389–416. In that essay I examine the question of whether Dr. Adams is obliged to obey the emergency conscription order—answering affirmatively, since obedience is here presumably a legitimate manifestation of a duty to participate in the protection of his nation against malicious threats from external sources. This question will not be posed in the current study, since it does not involve a coercive decision on Dr. Adams's part. Our interest in this section is in Dr. Adams as an agent of individual decisions for coercion.

5. Edmund D. Pellegrino and David C. Thomasma, *For the Patient's Good* (New York: Oxford University Press, 1988).

6. George Annas, "Control of Tuberculosis—the Law and the Public's Health," *New England Journal of Medicine* 328, no. 8 (1993): 585–88. One could argue that in most circumstances directly observed treatment actually serves the best interests of the patients who are coerced into receiving it. We will not address that issue here.

7. One might argue that there is no single overriding fundamental ethical principle, but rather several equally compelling fundamental principles that must be integrated in any decision. This approach is misleading, however, because it implies the existence of a single fundamental ethical principle of higher order—namely the principle that these lower-order "fundamental" principles should be integrated in such-and-such a way by the decision maker.

8. Immanuel Kant, *Foundations of the Metaphysics of Morals*, trans. Lewis White Beck (Indianapolis: Bobbs-Merrill, 1959), 37–42.

9. Analytic ethicists frequently lump teleology together with consequentialism. I have criticized this practice at length in several other essays and will not comment further about it here. Some species of consequentialism will integrate desires or other outcome-producing attributes into their account of the outcome (e.g., by defining the good as something like "the satisfaction of desires"). This strategy does not link them in any strong sense to teleologists, however, since for consequentialists the outcome-producing attribute has no intrinsic moral quality, is not susceptible to ethical criticism or revision (except, perhaps, insofar as it countervails other outcome-producing attributes of its type), and is not so much expressed as satisfied or extinguished in the outcome.

10. Trotter, "Loyalty in the Trenches."

11. It is possible for members of civil society to enact a polity without sharing common values—each participant having diverging reasons to approve the endeavor. In practice, however, such is not the case. Security from violence, for instance, enjoys consensus approval (despite differing degrees of emphasis). Not only does this value found agreement about the forensic and defensive duties of government, but it also founds the principle of permission (which is compelling just insofar as participating individuals and moral communities antecedently believe that using force requires an ethical rationale).

12. As I have argued at length elsewhere (contra Engelhardt), the principle of permission is not the transcendental condition for the possibility of a secular moral community and hence not part of a universal or galactic secular morality. It is, however, a necessary condition (and a fundamental principle) for any secular moral community that begins with the presumption that moral controversies should not be resolved by recourse to violence or force. Granted consensus that this will be the operative domain for secular morality (a consensus that would enlist Engelhardt because he thinks it is a conceptual truism, and enlist me because I think it is a common value), there is in practice not much difference between Engelhardt's version of

secular morality and mine (the remaining difference hinging mostly on my contention, versus Engelhardt, that many of the rules of property acquisition and ownership are contingencies that must themselves be resolved through an appeal to the principle of permission). Within a secular community bound by consensus that moral controversies should not be resolved by recourse to violence or force, there is good reason to extend a right not to be coerced without permission to those outside the community. This stance may increase the likelihood that external parties will refrain from using force against the polity or its citizens. It may also help evangelize others. And perhaps most important, the radical tolerance of indifference will run deeper within its own boundaries if it is respected outside these boundaries.

13. Trotter, *The Loyal Physician*.

14. Josiah Royce, *The Philosophy of Loyalty* (Nashville, Tenn.: Vanderbilt University Press, 1995 [1908]), 9.

Index

accountability, 104, 105–6

activism, 39, 129n24

Advisory Committee on Immunization Practices (ACIP), 61, 64

Agency for Healthcare Research and Quality (AHRQ), 35

aggregates, 108–10, 112–17

Aguirre, Benigno E., 130n35

AIDS/HIV, 122n30, 127n11

American College of Emergency Physicians, 4

Annas, George, 12–14, 77–79, 105

anthrax, viii, 81–82

anti-contagionists, 62

Aristotle, 118

assumptions: and disaster responses, 90–91; during September 11 attack, 85–87

Auf der Heide, Eric, 6, 104

Aum Shinrikyo, 89–91

authority, ix–x, 11, 72; federal vs. state vs. local, 75–83; and Incident Command System, 93–97; theories of, xii–xiii, 121n20; trust in, 13–14

autonomy, 5–6, 67–73

balance of powers, 34–35, 46

Baltimore, David, 144n46

Beauchamp, Dan, 23–24

Beauchamp, Tom L., 7–8, 10

biological agents, 80–83, 137n1

Biological-Chemical Agent Threat Classification, 81–83

bioterrorism, 10–13, 16, 119nn1–2, 127n11, 136n17

Bradshaw, Sandy, 84

Brandeis, Louis, 78

Brown, Michael, 139n4

Calhoun, John C., 49, 78, 129n29, 138n10

Carrol, Daniel, 132n47

catastrophes, 4–5, 65, 120n11

categorical imperative, 109–10

cell phones, 85–86, 102

Center for Law and the Public's Health (Georgetown and Johns Hopkins), 1

Centers for Disease Control and Prevention (CDC), 1, 10–11, 35, 77, 82

chemical agents, 89–93, 126n1, 137n1, 140n7

Cheney, Richard, 88

Childress, James F., 7–8, 10

Chisholm, Brock, 21–22

cholera, 62, 82

ciprofloxacin, 2, 120n6

civil rights, 14, 20, 105, 124n4

Clarke, Lee, 57–58

clinical medicine, x, 5–7, 55–56, 108–9, 113, 115

coercion, 1–14, 91; definitions of, vii, 7–10, 12, 122n25; guidelines for, ix, xiii–xiv, 104–18

Cohen, Joshua, 36

Cole, Dana, 141n21

Collins, Randall, 131n35

command and control, xiv, 95, 97, 120n11

common good, 16–20, 124n11, 125n17

common ground, 48, 50–51, 134n58

communitarians, 18–19

community, moral, 44, 74, 137n2

Compass, Edwin P., III, 65

compromise, 46–51

conditions model, 17–20, 124n11, 125n17

conscription, vii, 74, 83

consensus: moral, 38, 41, 48–49; overlapping, 37–40, 125nn11–12; weak, 133n53. See also rational consensus theory

consent, principle of, 44